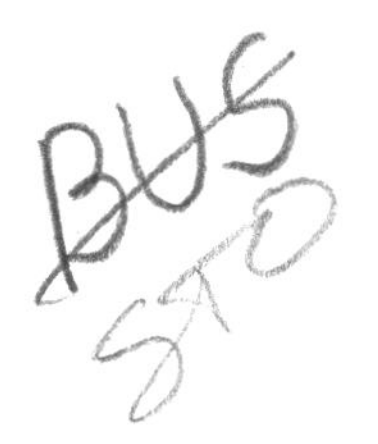

IS YOUR *AEROBICS* CLASS KILLING YOU?

IS YOUR *AEROBICS* CLASS KILLING YOU?

HOW TO MAKE DANCE EXERCISE SAFE & EFFECTIVE

DAVID Q. THOMAS, Ph.D.
&
NICKI E. RIPPEE, Ph.D.

a cappella books

Library of Congress Cataloging-in-Publication Data

Thomas, David Q.
Is your aerobics class killing you? : how to make exercise safe and effective / David Q. Thomas and Nicki E. Rippee.
p. cm.
Includes bibliographical references.
ISBN 1-55652-153-7 (pbk) : $11.95
1. Aerobic exercises—Safety measures. I. Rippee, Nicki E. II. Title.
RA781.15.T46 1992
613.7'1—dc20
92-31339
CIP

a cappella books
an imprint of Chicago Review Press, Incorporated

Editorial offices:
P.O. Box 380
Pennington, New Jersey 08534

Business/Sales offices:
814 N. Franklin St.
Chicago, IL 60610

All photos by Allan Gilmore

Models: Kim Lamb and Pam Robb of the Texas Club, Houston, TX

CONTENTS

I

Getting Started

II

III

Finishing Touches

I

GETTING STARTED

ONE

WHY SHOULD I READ THIS BOOK?

In 1990, aerobic exercise was the preferred way for 23.3 million Americans over the age of seven to keep in shape. And, every year, more and more people join an aerobic-fitness class. There's a reason aerobics is so popular: it's a fun way to tone up, lose a few extra pounds, and feel better about yourself. Exercising in a group can give you the motivation to keep on going even when you don't see immediate gains. And working out to music, a key element of many aerobics programs, takes you out of the gym and onto the dance floor!

But still, how can you be sure that the exercises you are asked to perform are truly safe? Who determines the qualifications of your aerobics leader and whether he or she is the best person to be leading an exercise class? What are the potential pitfalls and most common causes of injury, and how can they be avoided?

This book cannot provide all of the answers to your concerns about aerobic exercise, but it can give you the knowledge with which you can make your own judgments. By following some simple rules, you can determine the best exercise regime for yourself. Keeping your personal goals in mind is a far better way to build an exercise program than simply "keeping up with the Joneses."

Technically, aerobic exercise is any exercise that elevates your normal heart rate over an extended period of time, for at least twenty minutes, to work your cardiorespiratory (heart/lung) system. Dance-exercise classes have been called "aerobics" because they meet this criteria; however, they don't always provide a nonstop aerobic workout. Typically, a class breaks down into three major parts: a warmup, a workout, and a cool-down. And, during the workout itself, you may perform exercises that are not specifically "aerobic" in order to work certain muscle groups. So, in this book we address many types of exercise routines to cover everything you might encounter in your aerobics class.

Aerobics, aerobic dance, and dance exercise are but three of the many names used more or less interchangeably to describe the combination of exercise and dance movements set to music. We will use these terms in this book to describe the entire exercise program, from warmup through workout (the "true" aerobic section of the program) to cool-down, commonly found in most aerobic-dance classes.

Exercise can make you look and feel better. It can help you live longer and stay active throughout your life. However, exercise performed incorrectly can also be dangerous. We frequently sacrifice safety when exercising because we want to achieve the most benefit in the shortest period of time. We sometimes assume that because some exercise is good, more must be better. In addition, the exercises that we learn (especially those taught by individuals without a formal background in dance, physical education, physical therapy, or sportsmedicine) may not all be safe. Exercise in excess, and exercises that are performed incorrectly, can lead to injury. We can optimize the benefits of our workouts by being aware of exercises that require caution. We should also follow the general guidelines recommended for exercise participation.

WHY DO WE GET INJURED?

There is general agreement in the sportsmedicine community that dance-exercise injuries occur most frequently because of overtraining (trying to do too much) and/or poor technique. These injuries may be classified as sudden damage (it hurts right now) or gradual damage (it hurts in a couple of days/weeks/years). Repeated stress on a body part without allowing adequate time for its recovery (called *overuse*), or without adequate precautions for protecting areas of weakness, may result in sudden injury. Overuse is also frequently blamed for more persistent long-term injury. Specific exercises may increase your risk of injury.

Many of these exercises may be safe over a short period of time or for certain people. However, experts including Charles Corbin and Ruth Lindsey warn that the potential damage associated with these exercises is not always immediately apparent, surfaces only after a number of years, and may result in long-term damage.

WHAT SHOULD I BE AWARE OF?

There have been a number of recent articles focusing on exercises that may lead to injury. There has also been an accompanying debate as to why some exercises that have been practiced for years may appear to be safe but are now recognized as potentially harmful to some people. To explain this inconsistency, we need to look at who is performing the exercise, and how and why the exercise is being performed.

What Am I?

Exercisers in general can be classified into two groups: the athlete and the nonathlete. These two groups have different objectives for exercise, and each accepts a different level of risk. Athletes are sometimes called upon to assume risks inherent to the performance of their particular sport. They accept that their risk for injury is higher and train to minimize this risk. They also assume that the benefits of success outweigh the potential risk of injury. The nonathlete or recreational exerciser, however, has no need to assume unnecessary risk. The substantial benefits of exercise can be obtained through a lower-risk program.

Who Am I?

In the last decade and a half, dance exercise has grown rapidly in popularity, particularly among women. Individuals participating in dance exercise vary widely in background. James Garrick separates them into three groups. About 45 percent of the aerobic-dance population are thirty- to fifty-year-old women. For many of these women, aerobic dance is their only form of exercise. Another 45 percent are individuals who have added aerobics to a menu that already contains a variety of sport and recreational activities. Finally, about 10 percent of aerobic dancers are instructors. Exercise participation and its inherent risk varies from group to group. Each group has specific concerns that should be considered to make exercise safe and effective.

How Should I Exercise?

How you exercise is one such concern. According to Ruth Lindsey and Charles Corbin, there is a critical difference between group and individual exercise. Most recreational exercisers are part of a large class taught by a single instructor. In this setting, individualized instruction is not guaranteed and, in most cases, is impossible. Participants follow the instructor's lead and try to perform the same exercises at the same pace. In individualized instruction, an exercise specialist works one-on-one with you and exercises are designed for your unique physical make-up. In this situation, certain exercises that are not meant to be used in mass settings may be safely included to meet a specific purpose when the instructor has determined that they will not injure you.

Who Should Instruct Me?

Whether you are exercising in a large class or with a personal trainer, the importance of learning from a qualified instructor cannot be overemphasized. Intelligent consumers would not trust having their cars repaired by underqualified mechanics. Certainly your life and health are worth more than your car; choose your instructors on the basis of their qualifications. Chapter 2 includes further information on what to look for in an exercise program.

Why Am I Exercising?

Your reasons for exercising are important considerations in developing a safe and effective program. You may join a dance-exercise program for health reasons, to improve your self-image, or because it's more enjoyable to exercise in a group than alone. Although both the self-image and the social aspects are important, this book focuses on the health aspects of exercise. We know that regular exercise may act to lower your risk for the development of a number of degenerative diseases (heart attack, stroke, diabetes) and may act to retard the aging process. Maintaining an appropriate level of fitness also helps to prevent injury. However, whether you exercise for health benefits or for other reasons, it is vitally important that you select exercises that meet your needs while maintaining a lower risk of injury. In this way, your exercise program will not be interrupted by injury or slowed down by nagging aches and pains.

Why Do Some People Stop Exercising?

Exercise can provide many benefits. We need to remember, however, that it is not a cure-all for all people. According to Nancy Ryan, 50 percent of those who start a dance-exercise program dropout within six weeks. This low adherence rate may indicate that there is something wrong with their exercise programs or that other factors may be at work to prevent them from reaching their goals. Among the many reasons why people dropout are health-related reasons (injuries, illness, pregnancy, and low fitness levels) and intrinsic reasons (attitude, lack of motivation, poor self-image, lack of immediate gratification, lack of enjoyment, and discomfort). Extrinsic factors also play an important role for decreased adherence, such as class location, class time, frequency, intensity and duration, ineffective class leadership, and cost. Maintaining an exercise program takes time, discipline, and dedication. You must establish realistic goals and consistently put forth the effort required to achieve them. The results, however, should more than make up for any inconvenience.

WHAT DOES THIS BOOK HAVE TO OFFER ME?

This book will not attempt to present answers to all of your exercise problems. It will, however, focus on steps that you can take to ensure that your exercise program is safe and effective. Our intent is to identify those exercises that put you at risk and to suggest safer alternatives. We will begin with an analysis of the prescreening process, then take you through a typical aerobics class, from warmup, through workouts for each area of the body, to cooling-down.

The information presented will be of value to the beginner as well as the advanced exerciser and even the aerobics instructor. Most of the exercises in this book are frequently performed in aerobic-dance classes and in the warmup for other types of physical activity or sport. In preparing this book, we have made an extensive study of the literature on aerobics, dance, and sportsmedicine. A complete list of dance-exercise participants, teachers, researchers, and physicians who have investigated these issues is given in the reference list and bibliography at the end of the book.

THE BOTTOM LINE!

Remember that exercise must not only be effective, it must also be safe. Not all of the exercises listed as risky in this book will injure everyone; however, they have the potential to increase your chance of injury. In many cases safer exercises are available, so why take a chance? Keep in mind that while you may have been doing many of these exercises for years, they have the potential for causing gradual injury that may show up twenty years down the road. According to James Garrick, "Even though aerobic dance appears less hazardous than most of the fitness alternatives such as running and tennis, it obviously can be made even safer." Our goal will be to identify the safest possible routines to optimize your enjoyment, while steering clear of hazardous exercise.

TWO

WHAT SHOULD I LOOK FOR IN AN AEROBICS CLASS?

Getting the Most for Your Money

Finding an aerobics class to suit your needs can be difficult. There are many different types of dance-exercise workouts available, ranging from classes designed to work specific areas of the body, to those for overall fitness, to exercise videos, to television shows. Selecting the right class is a very important part of ensuring that your objectives are met. This chapter gives a brief overview of what to look for in an instructor and the key differences among the various aerobics classes. We will also discuss exercise concerns for people of various ages and for the pregnant exerciser.

EVALUATING AN AEROBICS INSTRUCTOR

When you pay to participate in an aerobics class or join a health club, you have the right to expect quality instruction. Anything less should not be acceptable and may even be dangerous. How then can you determine that you are getting the most for your money?

Beauty or Brains?

The most important determinant as to whether you receive the safest and most effective instruction is the quality of your exercise leader. The exercise leader's primary purpose is to provide you with high-quality instruction and useful information that will make you a more informed exerciser. Finding a good instructor is not difficult if you know what to look for. By following the dos and don'ts listed below, you will increase the likelihood that you are getting the best instruction available.

Dos and Don'ts in Selecting an Aerobics Class

Don't

- Be fooled by looks alone. Our looks are heavily influenced by our genetics. Looking good does not necessarily correlate with advanced knowledge in how to effectively teach someone how to exercise. We all know people who look great but who know little about how to exercise, let alone how to teach someone else to exercise. On the other hand, don't entirely disregard someone because they are good-looking. (After all, there are some of us with good looks and brains; just check the mirror.) Don't judge the book by its cover: find out what your instructor knows. If you're not entirely satisfied, find another instructor.
- Accept leadership from someone who is primarily there to sell memberships. Many facilities hire individuals to sell memberships and increase company profit. You want instructors who have as their priority leading you through a safe and effective workout.
- Get sold on celebrity status. Famous people are not necessarily more knowledgeable people. There are numerous exercise videos put out by celebrities that contain misinformation and exercises that are dangerous.
- Play follow the leader. Exercise instructors probably have a different level of fitness than you do and are performing at a pace that is comfortable for them. Your leader should encourage you to set your own pace and to alter the exercises to best suit your needs. Dance exercise is not competitive.

Do

- Check on the instructors' qualifications. Do they have degrees from accredited institutions in physical education or fitness? Can they tell a *tibia* from a *femur*? Have they studied anatomy and physiology? Remember, it's important to find instructors who know what they are doing. Would you select a physician who never went to medical school?

- Make sure that your instructor is certified from a nationally recognized association. The three best organizations are the American College of Sports Medicine (ACSM), the American Council on Exercise (ACE, formerly the International Dance Exercise Association or IDEA), and the American Fitness and Aerobics Association (AFAA). Beware! There are many fly-by-night certification agencies that will certify anyone with a pulse and an address who can afford the application fee.
- Find someone who is energetic and motivational. You will, after all, have to look at and listen to this person for twenty to sixty minutes several times a week. And we all can use a motivational boost every now and then.
- Find someone who includes an educational component in every class. You should understand what you are doing and why you are doing it. Additionally, the instructor should tell you how to correctly perform the exercise and how to modify it to meet your individual needs and fitness level.
- Find leaders who focus on you and not themselves. You are not paying for their workout.
- Get your physician's clearance before participating in an aerobics class. It may take extra time and effort on your part, but the consequences may be severe if you don't take this necessary precaution.
- Find someone who frequently reminds you to monitor your level of exertion. You should be encouraged to check your intensity (usually by monitoring your pulse) at least every ten minutes.
- Find someone who will not allow you to participate without a proper warmup and who will not allow you to leave without a proper cool-down. Warming-up and cooling-down are crucial to making sure that your program is both safe and effective.

Choosing an Aerobics Class

"Aerobics" is a catchall term applied to many different types of exercise, some involving dance movements, some not. Aerobics classes are offered everywhere, from local YM/YWCAs, night schools, and dance studios to specialized aerobic studios, health clubs, and college classes. It would be wise to visit a class at least once before signing up. Many studios offer a free trial visit, or the option of enrolling for a few classes before making you sign on the dotted line. You don't want to spend a large sum of money buying a year's worth of aerobics classes only to discover that the instructor, the other exercisers, a poorly designed exercise regime, or an uncomfortably crowded space makes it impossible for you to enjoy your workout.

A key component in any dance-exercise class is the use of musical accompaniment, usually emphasizing today's top-forty hits. However, there are now classes drawing on all types of music, from heavy metal to jazz to world music to light classics. You should ask whether you'll be sweatin' to the classics or bumping and grinding to rap. Obviously, different people have different musical likes and dislikes.

Finally, the aerobics field is becoming increasingly specialized. There are now classes just for kids, for teens, adults, and senior citizens. Some may enjoy working out with other people in their own age group, while others may prefer to workout in a mixed class. Also, there are classes just for women, just for pregnant women, and singles-only classes; there are high-intensity, low-intensity, and mixed-intensity workouts; there are step-aerobics and power workouts; there's even Afro-Aerobics and country-and-western aerobics. Again, choose an environment that will make you comfortable.

TYPES OF AEROBICS CLASSES

Aerobics classes combine choreographed movements with group calisthenics designed to enhance overall fitness. Aerobics programs that feature a greater emphasis on group calisthenics are usually found in health clubs or YM/YWCAs. They are popular because the steps are easy to follow, allowing beginners who may not feel that they are great dancers to participate. They can be adapted to fit any musical taste and attract the largest number of male participants.

Jackie Sorenson founded one of the first forms of group dance-exercise, Aerobic Dance, in 1969. Sorenson's brand of aerobics is based on choreographed patterns of dance movements. The workout is primarily designed to work the cardiovascular system, but also includes segments of floor exercises and flexibility work. Unlike the calisthenic-oriented classes, Aerobic Dance is most popular among those with some dance training, appealing more strongly to women and younger exercisers.

Jazzercise is another form of aerobics and was developed by Judy Sheppard Missett. Like Aerobic Dance, Jazzercise is oriented toward dance movement and is more popular among women than men. Its original focus was on muscle-group work and the incorporation of new dance trends. Jazzercise is highly choreographed and uses many dance steps to give you an aerobic workout. Although you don't have to be a dancer to participate in either Aerobic Dance or Jazzercise, dance steps make up a significant portion of the class and add versatility, fun, and variety to exercise.

Site-specific exercise classes are designed to work on one part of your body or one area of fitness. "Stretch and tone" classes increase flexibility and muscular strength and endurance, but are not designed to increase cardiovascular endurance. Abdominal workouts are designed to tone the abdominal muscles and do little else for other areas of the body. When participating in these classes, keep in mind the purpose of the class and remember that there is no such thing as "spot reducing" site-specific fat. All the side leg raises in the world won't give you "thin thighs"!

Classes are also named for the impact associated with their performance. Low-impact, variable-impact, and high-impact aerobic classes are named for the kinds of movements you make. They are all designed for aerobic work, so don't confuse these with the terms low and high intensity that refer to how hard you work. Low-impact aerobics can offer a high-intensity workout.

Most of the early aerobics classes featured high-impact movements. High-impact aerobics incorporate movements where both feet are occasionally off the floor at the same time, including jumping jacks, jogging, and small jumps or hops (as in a knee lift when you hop on the supporting foot as you raise the knee of your other leg). The music is normally between 140 and 180 beats per minute (bpm). Injuries in high-impact classes seem to be related primarily to overuse, poor footwear, and hard exercise surfaces.

Low-impact classes are designed to lessen the impact stress on the body. One foot is kept on the ground at all times, so you won't be jogging or jumping. Instead, marching, traveling moves across the floor, and upper-body work are used to give you a complete workout with more arm movement than is found in high-impact aerobics. The music used in these classes has a slower tempo (usually between 125 and 140 bpm). This type of exercise is as effective as high-impact aerobics for improving cardiovascular fitness, muscular strength, and endurance and increasing your use of fat as a fuel source. Low-impact classes are useful for all fitness levels and are particularly appropriate if you want to avoid the jarring activity of jogging or high-impact exercises.

Don't be misled into the belief that low-impact aerobics are not without risk. It was first thought that a shift to low-impact aerobics would decrease the probability of injury. However, it seems that the potential for injury in both high- and low-impact aerobics is similar, although frequently different areas of the body may be injured. As with all exercise injury, prevention lies in practicing proper exercise technique and following recommended exercise guidelines and procedures.

Variable-impact classes use both low- and high-impact movements. The tempo of the music varies according to the movement performed, but should always be slow enough to allow you to maintain good body alignment and mechanics.

GETTING A STEP UP ON FITNESS

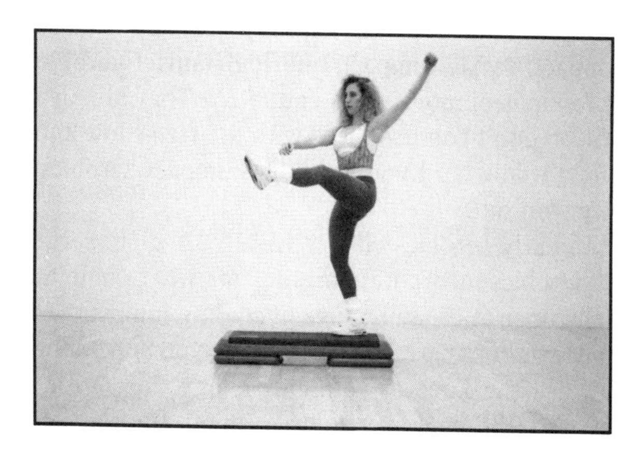

The latest rage in the fitness industry is step aerobics. This relatively new trend takes an old practice of stepping as a form of exercise and modifies it to fit a dance-aerobics setting. Step training involves using a variety of step combinations on benches ranging in height from six to twelve inches. These step combinations are choreographed to music. Step training is popular because the moves are easier to learn than those in regular aerobics routines, while providing a greater exercise workload. Preliminary research into this new training method indicates that you can receive cardiovascular benefits similar to walking and jogging with less impact on your joints. The addition of hand weights can further increase workload, making step aerobics popular for those who feel they may not be getting enough out of aerobic dance. Additionally, the perception that step training places particular emphasis on exercising the thighs and buttocks attracts others to this new fitness trend.

When selecting a step-training class, the bottom line is finding a good instructor who helps you to modify the exercise to meet your individual needs and goals. There have been some questions as to whether step training is recommended for everyone. We suggest that, as with all exercise, you check with your physician before trying any new exercise program. Additionally, pay attention to your body's response to the exercise. Your body will inform you if you are not responding properly. More research is necessary before conclusions about the safety of repeated step training is known, but there have been some reports of increased injuries to the knee, ankle, and lower back. At this point in time, step training seems to be a functional, alternative method of improving your fitness. Time will tell if it is as safe as other methods.

GETTING OFF ON THE RIGHT FOOT

The first step in any aerobics program is to purchase shoes that will maximize the benefits of your workout while minimizing the risk of injury. Proper footwear provides stability and cushioning while preventing slippage, allowing mobility while providing for comfort.

How Do You Know Which Shoe Is Right for You?

There are some general guidelines to follow when purchasing shoes specifically for use in aerobic dance. Consider your level of participation. If you participate in aerobic dance two or three times per week for an hour or so each time, then you will need a shoe made specifically for aerobics rather than a cross-training shoe. If you are exercising more than five hours per week, you will need to buy new shoes at least three times per year.

When choosing a shoe, get the right fit. Everyone's foot is different, so do not pick a shoe based on what the instructor or a friend wears. Different brands of shoes are made with different lasts (the mold on which the shoe is shaped) and will fit each individual foot differently. For example, Adidas shoes are made on a narrow last, while New Balance makes shoes in a variety of widths. Buy your shoes later in the day when your feet are slightly swollen; this will most closely approximate an exercise situation. Make sure that the toe box is roomy; a half-inch space between the longest toe and the end of the shoe is recommended. This is important because your foot will flatten out when landing from a jump. Choose a shoe that fits the shape of your foot (C-curved or straight). Try on several brands and pairs.

Glenn Ocker made an extensive study of aerobic shoes. He noted that lateral stability is of particular importance for your safety, which is provided by straps, heel counters, flexible outer soles, sole width, and the rigidity of the upper part of the shoe.

Lateral straps are panels across the widest part of the shoe. They help to provide protection from knee or ankle injuries. Typically they run from the outer sole region and connect to the lacing. They should be located at the ball of the foot.

Heel counters are a plastic or cardboard surface around the heel. Your shoe must have them to support your heels properly, and they must be rigid. They keep the heels centered during impact.

Flexed or notched outer soles help the foot bend freely. You should look for reduced patterning at the ball of the foot, a thinner outer sole, or a groove or different material at the notch that allows for easier foot flexion.

The outer soles should extend about a quarter-inch wider than the heel counter. Soles that are flared (or platformed) too wide (as in a running shoe) may cause injury by catching on the floor when you are performing lateral movements.

Make sure that the sole is wide enough for your foot. The side of your foot should not hang over the sole of the shoe. Check to see that the upper part of the shoe is made of firm-grained leather so that it will resist stretching over time.

Shock absorbency under the ball of the foot is also important. Your shoe may have a different color or texture in the sole, indicating that special impact-absorbing material has been added to protect your foot. However, be careful of gimmicks from the manufacturer. The added color may do nothing more than attract the eye.

Comfort and some injury protection is crucial. You should look for a liner that does not trap heat or chafe. For this reason, you should avoid terry-cloth or nylon liners. A good liner will absorb moisture and reduce friction. Look for ventilation holes to keep your foot cool and for a well-padded tongue for comfort and protection.

The shoe's lacing system should feature holes cut in the leather to allow adjusting the tension of the laces for an individualized fit. Shoes with variable-width lacing will provide some adjustment for different feet. Avoid shoes with metal D-ring lacing; this spreads the tension evenly over the foot so that you cannot control tension in different spots. Choose shoes without velcro or strap fasteners on the arch; they are O.K. for high-top sneakers to secure the lacing, but they do not add support to low-cut aerobic shoes.

Look for a high, well-cushioned arch and for a notch cut out of the back of the heel area to protect the Achilles tendon in high-, mid-, or three-quarter-cut shoes.

In summary, remember that good shoes are designed to protect you from injury and keep you exercising. A good shoe provides stability; when your foot comes down to the floor, you must have a firm base with good balance. The shoe should also provide support for your foot and ankle and good shock-absorbing qualities. You may want to ask about the materials used in the sole and how they provide good shock absorption. The shoe needs to be flexible at the ball of the foot because of the nature of aerobic dance. Many steps require you to land on the ball of the foot first, and the shoe needs to bend easily where your foot bends.

When shopping for your shoes, be sure to try on several styles and brands; try a few steps in each pair, then pick the pair that feels best to you. Remember, if a shoe hurts in the store, it will probably hurt in class. But be careful of the shoe that feels like your house slippers; it won't meet the criteria for stability and shock absorption. There are many good shoes on the market and, by following our recommendations, you shouldn't go wrong.

Finally, never participate in an aerobics class barefoot or in stockinged feet. If you do, you risk injuring your feet or lower legs. Your feet alone are not designed to withstand the shocks of a dance-exercise workout.

WHAT IS THE BEST SURFACE TO EXERCISE ON?

The surface on which you exercise will also affect the safety of your exercise program. As with shoes, a good surface allows for shock absorption and prevents slippage. Generally, the recommended surface across the aerobic-dance industry is a spring-loaded wooden floor such as that found in most gymnasiums. If a surface is too hard (concrete or carpet over concrete) your risk for stress fracture and overuse injury increases. If the surface is too soft, muscle imbalance and joint injury potentially become a problem.

VIDEOS AND BOOKS

Exercise videos, television shows, and books can play an important role in augmenting your aerobics classes. However, not everything you see in a video or read in an exercise book will suit your needs or provide an injury-free workout. In fact, a significant amount of material on the market borders on being downright dangerous. It is up to you to use your judgment to make sure that whatever exercise program you follow meets your goals.

There are far too many videos and books available on the market for us to review in this book. But, we suggest that you judge the book or video by content rather than by presentation. You must look further than the cover or packaging to determine if it is right for you. Look to see who is responsible for the information presented. This means looking beyond the typical celebrity or "body beautiful" who presents the information to the person who provides the expert advice. Then ask, what qualifies that person to give advice on exercise? Is he or she a physician with training in sportsmedicine or in physical education? Does the advice make sense? Lack of expert guidance is usually a very good indicator that a video or book is not a good one. Additionally, check to see if the video or book has the support or backing of established organizations of exercise professionals (ACSM, ACE, AAHPERD, AFAA).

Examine the claims made by the book or video. If they sound too good to be true, they usually are. Exercise is based on firmly established scientific principles. We know that exercise can make you be the best that you can be if you are willing to work for it. But it will not turn you into someone you are not and will not bring about miraculous changes. If the book or video recommends something that feels bad or seems wrong, don't do it. Check to see if the established guidelines for exercise participation are followed as presented in this book, and never follow an exercise program without first checking with your physician.

Finally, remember that we are all different physically and we all have different goals and objectives. Therefore, no book or video designed for the mass market is perfect for everyone. You will have to modify any exercise program to suit your own needs.

EXERCISE AND AGE

People of any age can enjoy the benefits of exercise. Exercise is quite safe if the proper principles are followed. Generally, the exercise response will be similar across the entire age spectrum. A healthy individual of any age who practices the accepted procedures for exercise participation should not have a problem. There are, however, certain considerations that must be kept in mind for the very young and the very old.

Children

It is important for elementary school-age children to have opportunities to be active in developmentally appropriate activities. Exercise programs for children need to be led by trained individuals who understand their maturational level and interests. These programs should address the health-related components of exercise in a fun way. For example, adults may be willing to run laps to improve the cardiovascular system, but for children an aerobic game would provide the same benefit while standing a better chance of holding their interest. Children are much more likely to play a fun game that is specifically designed for them than to perform rigidly structured exercise. We want children to enjoy physical activity and establish good exercise habits so that they will continue to exercise as adults.

One special consideration for children is their inability to regulate their temperature as efficiently as adults. They have more difficulty cooling-down than adults, so they need to drink plenty of water before, during, and after activity. We must also remember that children are not little adults. Their bones and muscles are not mature and extra caution is required when performing load-bearing exercises. Specific guidelines are available from the International Athletics Association Federation (IAAF) Medical Committee and the National Strength and Conditioning Association for long-distance running and weight training.

Older Populations

Being physically active as senior citizens is particularly important to maintain health, a better quality of life, and independent living. Some research suggests that 50 percent of aging decline is preventable through a positive lifestyle, including regular exercise. Active women and men are physiologically ten to twenty years younger than their sedentary peers. And the good news is that older people can experience the benefits of exercise at any age, even if they have been inactive most of their lives.

Older people will have different exercise needs, depending on their overall health, experience, and the type of exercise that they enjoy. Some older people may need to limit themselves to lower-impact activities such as walking or swimming, while others can still enjoy activities such as tennis and jogging. The maintenance of mobility, strength, and flexibility are particularly important for older persons. Aerobic exercise can have a positive effect on your blood pressure, reducing body fat and cholesterol, and maintaining good reaction time.

Like the very young, it is very important for older exercisers to drink plenty of water. Temperature-regulation problems associated with poorer circulation require increased consumption of fluids. Remember that thirst is not an adequate indicator of the need for water and usually indicates that dehydration has already set in. It is important to drink water before feeling thirsty. Anyone who has difficulty cooling-down should also exercise at relatively cool times of the day or in a cool exercise room.

Keeping fit can make the difference between continued independent living and a life in a full-time health-care facility. Working with an exercise leader who follows established exercise principles, creates a program that meets your individual needs and limitations, and follows physician recommendations will make for a balanced and enjoyable program.

Pregnancy

Is exercise appropriate during pregnancy? This is a difficult question to answer for all women. As in the general population, no two pregnant women are exactly the same, so all guidelines will have to be modified to meet your individual needs.

The first step is to consult with your physician. If you have not been on a regular exercise program, you should not start one when pregnant. However, with certain modifications, most women can continue an exercise program. Different organizations, such as the American College of Obstetricians and Gynecologists (ACOG), have published guidelines for exercise by pregnant women. Many women feel that these guidelines tend to be conservative, but they reflect the perception that it is better to experience deconditioning than to jeopardize the health and welfare of the mother or child.

The benefits of exercise for pregnant women are improved muscle tone, added strength, added endurance, decreased lower-back pain, increased energy, a positive mood, and improved self-image. Most doctors recommend mild to moderate physical activity, but you need to be aware of your body's response to pregnancy and follow the guidelines for safe exercise. Regular exercise is safer than sporadic exercise, so exercise at least three times a week. The ACOG guidelines recommend no more than fifteen minutes of aerobic exercise because the body's core temperature increases after twenty minutes. This can be potentially dangerous to the fetus because it has no capacity for cooling. You also should not exercise under very hot, humid conditions or in poorly ventilated exercise rooms.

You should take in enough calories to meet the extra needs of the pregnancy and exercise, and drink water before, during, and after a workout to avoid becoming dehydrated. Pregnant women are at a greater risk than other exercisers for dehydration, which can cause premature labor, so plenty of water, whether or not you feel thirsty, is a must. The ACOG recommends that your heart rate not exceed 140 beats per minute due to potential disruptions in blood flow to the fetus. Do not exercise to the point of exhaustion or chronic fatigue (feeling tired for more than an hour after exercise). Precede exercise with an easy ten-minute warmup and follow exercise with a five- to ten-minute cool-down until your heart rate is below 100 beats per minute.

You may need to discontinue prolonged exercises performed on your back, particularly after the fourth month. Your enlarged uterus can interfere with the circulation of your blood to the fetus and its return to your heart. If you become dizzy, short of breath, nauseous, or feel tingling in your lower limbs while exercising on your back, roll onto your left side and remain in that position until the discomfort passes. If this condition recurs, you should avoid the position or remain on your back for very short periods of time. Joints, ligaments, and tendons become more lax during pregnancy and therefore are more prone to injury, so avoid activities that require jumping, jarring motions, or rapid changes in direction. If an activity becomes uncomfortable due to joint instability, modify or stop this activity. If you experience any unusual symptoms such as bleeding, cramping, faintness, elevated blood pressure, dizziness, or joint pain, stop exercising and consult your doctor immediately.

The ACOG guidelines include some conditions under which no exercise should be done, so it is extremely important to check with your doctor if you plan on exercising when pregnant. Pregnant women who have suffered from two or more miscarriages, or who have heart disease, vaginal bleeding, a multiple pregnancy, a weak cervix, ruptured membranes, misplaced placenta, or premature labor should not participate in an exercise program.

When choosing an activity, consider your prepregnancy fitness and activity level and do not try to exceed it. Some lower-impact activities may be appropriate such as low-impact aerobics, stationary rowing, swimming, stair stepping, water aerobics, walking, or stationary cycling. Find an activity you enjoy because one of the most consistent benefits of exercise during pregnancy is psychological. These are but a brief summary of guidelines for exercise during pregnancy. Be sure to ask your doctor for further advice, work with an exercise instructor trained in exercise and pregnancy, and enjoy the benefits.

MEN AND WOMEN

Men and women generally respond to exercise in the same way. Recent studies suggest that there is more variability within either population than between the sexes regarding exercise response. Although traditionally more women that men participate in dance-exercise classes, they can both benefit from this excellent form of exercise.

There are some structural differences between men and women that can influence their exercise response. Men typically can achieve higher levels of aerobic fitness in terms of absolute measurements of oxygen consumption, due to their larger lung capacity, and they can achieve greater levels of strength due to hormonal and size differences. However, women can achieve similar levels of aerobic fitness in proportion to their body size, and also have been known to achieve significant gains in strength. Although your commitment to exercise, your genetic background, and your gender will have some impact on your response to exercise, everyone can benefit from a regular exercise program.

THREE

WHAT SHOULD I DO WHEN STARTING AN EXERCISE PROGRAM?

Prescreening

Although we all want to jump right into an aerobics program once we have made the commitment to exercise, caution must take precedence over enthusiasm if we want to get the most out of it. An important guideline to ensure safe and effective exercise is proper prescreening. Experts generally agree that exercise is a safe activity for most individuals. However, according to the American College of Sports Medicine, everyone should have some prescreening prior to starting an exercise program or taking an exercise test.

WHY SHOULD I BE PRESCREENED?

Prescreening prior to your participation in an exercise program can predict potential problems and eliminate or lower your risk. A fitness program cannot be considered either safe or effective without these factors being considered. A secondary objective of prescreening is to provide baseline information on initial fitness levels. This information can be used to evaluate your progress as well as the effectiveness of your exercise program.

Prescreening should involve a partnership between you, your physician, and your exercise leader. All three are critical to making the program a success, and they all need to be aware of any potential risks or problems. Each one plays an important and different role in successful exercise participation. Your physician diagnoses disease or injury, sets guidelines for an exercise program, and determines whether you are healthy enough to exercise. Your exercise leader should safely guide you through the exercise program and act as a consultant regarding it. You must then take the ultimate responsibility for fully implementing the plan and honestly reporting any abnormal symptoms.

WHAT SHOULD I BE PRESCREENED FOR?

The prescreening process typically includes a medical exam, a health-history appraisal, and a fitness evaluation. Depending on the type of exercise program that you wish to participate in, your exercise leader may be involved in all or part of the prescreening process. In any case, your exercise leader must be informed of, and have access to, the results of all information gathered during the prescreening.

THE MEDICAL EXAM

The American College of Sports Medicine suggests that the depth of your medical screening should be based upon your age, health status, test availability, and exercise plan. Because regular physical exams are an important part of ensuring good health and fitness, prescreening should always begin with a consultation with your physician, who will know about any pre-existing limitations to your exercise participation. You should consult your doctor prior to beginning an exercise program or prior to making any significant increase in your exercise regimen, and be prepared to ask specific exercise-related health questions, focusing on:

1. Your limitations for exercise. Do you have any conditions that would preclude exercise? Are there any limits to the types of exercises that you can perform?
2. The effects of any medications that you may be taking (both prescription and over-the-counter) on your response to exercise.

3. The effect of any injuries, past or present, on your exercise capabilities.

In addition to the exam by your physician, your exercise instructor should gather data on injury, medication, disease, family history, coronary-artery disease risk, blood pressure, and information regarding your primary physician and health-care provider (health insurance company). In addition, your exercise history, nutritional history, and informed consent should be obtained.

Your medical history is important because it allows your exercise instructor to be sure that the exercises that are included in the routine are safe for you. Old and new injuries should be analyzed because, once an injury has occurred, the site is predisposed to further injury. Over-the-counter and prescription medications that you are using may affect your body's response and adaptation to exercise. For instance, diet pills may act as stimulants that raise your resting and exercise heart rates. This may lead to cardiovascular stress that is beyond the limits that can be safely tolerated, increasing your risk of experiencing a cardiac event. Your physician, exercise leader, and you must be aware of the contraindications and side effects of all medications.

Your exercise leader also needs to know if you are ill. You should not exercise when you're sick, because it may prolong your illness and increase the stress on your body, resulting in further medical complications. In addition, exercise instructors should be aware of any diseases or symptoms that you may have. This will allow them to be better prepared to deal with any emergency, should one occur. These signs or symptoms are also invaluable when modifying an exercise program.

The results of the Framingham Heart Study indicate that family history plays a major role in your risk for disease. (This ongoing research project has followed the inhabitants of Framingham, Massachusetts, since the 1950s to determine what risk factors are associated with early death and disease.) It is also well known that genetics are a major factor in determining your potential for exercise and sport performance. For these reasons, your exercise leader must gather information on your family history, including an analysis of the coronary-artery disease risk factors that you have. These factors can be used to predict your risk of dying prematurely from a heart attack. The major risk factors associated with the development of cardiovascular disease are: high blood pressure, smoking, high cholesterol levels, inactivity, obesity, stress, age, gender, race, diabetes, and family history.

Because approximately 2 percent of our population is classified as hypertensive (having chronically elevated blood pressure), and because uncontrolled hypertension may lead to severe conditions when combined with the stress of exercise, your prescreening process should also include an assessment of your blood pressure. Normal blood pressure response falls into the range of 120 to 140 over 70 to 90. However, it is important to remember that blood pressure is dependent on your age and size. Unusual blood pressure readings should be rechecked and your physician consulted if these unusual readings persist.

THE HEALTH HISTORY

Your initial health history may or may not be obtained by your exercise instructor; it should, however, be reviewed by your instructor. According to L. Kent Smith, a complete health appraisal should include an analysis of health behaviors (diet, exercise, smoking, stress), health history (family history, personal history), and a physiologic appraisal (blood pressure, diabetes, blood fats, body composition). When you enter into an exercise class, it is your instructor's responsibility to provide further prescreening. This is one way of determining whether you have a good instructor. No one should enter into an exercise situation without being prescreened. This is important not only to protect your instructor from legal liability but also for your health and welfare.

Nutrition

Because we are what we eat, and because we cannot improve our fitness and health without proper nutrition, your prescreening process should also include your nutritional history. No matter how much you exercise, there are certain nutrients that must be consumed. These include: carbohydrates, the primary source of energy in high-intensity exercise; fats, the primary source of energy in long-duration and low-to-moderate intensity exercise; and protein, the key building block for muscular development. It is generally recommended that complex carbohydrates make up the largest portion of your diet. You should be consuming 55 to 65 percent carbohydrates, 20 to 30 percent fat, and 10 to 15 percent protein, focusing your diet on grains, fruits, vegetables, and legumes. If you eat meat, it should be lean and consumed in modest quantities. If you choose not to consume meat, you must be very careful to supplement your diet to ensure that you obtain the essential amino acids found in meat from other

food sources. Because this sometimes can be difficult, it is recomm
that you consult with a registered dietitian or your physician.

Contrary to popular belief, you don't need to increase your consumption of protein before exercising. As we exercise, we eat more (we also use more energy, so less is stored as fat), ensuring that our diet has an adequate amount of protein. In fact, too much protein can lead to dehydration and potential liver and kidney damage. Protein supplements should not be taken without first consulting your physician.

Vitamins and minerals are important nutrients found in most of the food that we eat. Eating a well-balanced diet will ensure that these needs are met. Supplementation of vitamins and minerals is generally not needed or recommended. If, however, you suspect that you are not eating a well-balanced diet, you should have your diet analyzed by a registered dietitian. Taking multivitamins and mineral supplements will only reduce the thickness of your wallet and may lead to physiological damage (hypervitaminosis and liver and kidney damage). In addition, a shotgun approach to supplementation is unwise. If your body needs medication, you don't take every type of medicine found in the drugstore. Use only the vitamins that your body needs in the doses recommended by a registered dietitian or physician.

The Fitness Assessment: Informed Consent

Informed consent should be obtained from all exercise participants. This ensures that you are aware of the potential risks and benefits associated with your exercise program, and that all of your questions have been answered to your satisfaction. By signing an informed consent form, you indicate that you are participating voluntarily. Unlike a waiver or release, the informed consent does not remove your instructor's or the exercise studio's liability for the safety of your exercise program. A waiver or release form is designed to protect the facility or instructor and has as its primary purpose removing their legal liability. The informed consent protects both you and your instructor. The informed-consent form is designed to ensure that your rights are maintained and that your instructor is protected.

Exercise History

A crucial component of your prescreening process is your exercise history. To optimize the benefits of an exercise program, you should know your current fitness status. Your instructor can then recommend the correct amount of exercise for optimal benefit, safety, and results. In addition, this information can be used to select activities that you enjoy. To ensure that a program is both safe and effective, you will need to modify your workout to suit your physical needs; the information gathered in an exercise history may be used as a starting point in this process.

Other Prescreening Tests

Prescreening can involve many different kinds of assessments. These may include measures of body composition (percent body fat), muscular strength, muscular endurance, flexibility, and cardiovascular fitness. The American College of Sports Medicine recommends that, if you are apparently healthy and under the age of forty-five, you do not require a maximal stress test. If you are over the age of forty-five, classified as at higher risk, or suffering from a disease, you should participate in an exercise stress test, preferably under the supervision of your physician.

SUMMARY

Testing for testing's sake is not a valid reason for prescreening; what is done with the prescreening results is as important as the process itself. Larry Gettman suggests that the results can be used to diagnose your strengths and weaknesses, monitor your achievement of individual goals, for educational purposes, motivation, and program evaluation. There is no valid excuse, either legally or ethically, for not prescreening. As an exercise consumer, you should demand it, and as an exercise leader, you should require it.

II

HOW DO I AVOID INJURY ?

DECISIONS, DECISIONS!

In all exercise situations, we make a choice of selecting activities to stress our bodies with the hope of attaining optimal fitness. This choice includes a decision to accept a certain level of risk in return for the benefits associated with performance of the activity. However, many of the activities that we have been taught put us under unacceptable levels of risk. There are a number of exercises that need to be eliminated from use, others that need to be modified, and others that may not cause immediate harm but which have safer alternatives. Peter and Lorna Francis define contraindicated exercises as those that place excessive stress on the anatomical structures of the human body. This part of the book will present these exercises and recommend safer alternatives if they exist.

HOW CAN SOME EXERCISES BE DANGEROUS?

Carol Goodman explains that there are several common exercise movements that put you at risk, particularly hyperflexion (bending too much) and hyperextension (straightening too much). Flexion is defined as moving two body segments toward each other. For example, when lifting a glass up to the mouth, the elbow is in a state of flexion. Extension is defined as moving two body segments away from each other. When lowering the glass back to the table, the elbow is moving in extension. Normal flexion and extension rarely cause problems. However, too much flexion and too much extension, especially when performed with bouncing movement or with additional weight, can lead to injury. When these positions are taken to the extreme, your risk of injury increases significantly.

Hyperflexion and hyperextension in a controlled movement with little or no additional load may not cause injury. The potential for injury becomes greatest when these movements shift the stress of maintaining the position from the muscles to the ligaments (connective tissues that attach bone to bone) and joints in positions of weakness. Additional stress caused by supporting the entire body weight, by using arm and ankle weights, by bouncing (ballistic movement), or by pushing off against a supporting surface can aggravate this problem. When the forces and torques (rotary equivalent of force) of this additional stress must be counteracted by the ligaments and cartilage, the risk for injury is increased. This may lead to overstretching in the ligament, cartilage injury, or herniation and rupture of the vertebral discs. In addition, the muscles and tendons (connective tissue that attaches muscle to bone) are put at an increased risk of strain.

HOW DO THESE INJURIES OCCUR?

According to Ruth Lindsey and Charles Corbin, many injuries caused by these exercises are gradual in nature; that is, they don't show up immediately, but build up over a period of years. When the injury surfaces later in life, its cause is frequently misdiagnosed and is commonly attributed to the aging process. Your lack of awareness of the injury can aggravate the situation. The fact that you don't feel sudden sharp pain may give you a false sense of security. In turn, this may lead you to continue the activity, resulting in further injury.

Another frequent cause of aerobic-dance injury, especially among instructors, is overuse. Overuse injuries occur when a movement is repeated over and over without the required resting period between activities. In addition, if the exercise or activity is not performed correctly, it may cause microtraumas (mini-injuries) that, over time, can lead to more significant injury. Microtraumas are minute tears in the muscle or connective tissue and are usually caused by friction or repeated strain; Marjorie Albohm labels this as the primary cause of aerobic-dance injury.

As you repeat an exercise, there is a tendency to allow incorrect movements to occur, due either to fatigue or to lack of skill. Ruth Lindsey and Charles Corbin warn us that "the odds of performing a hazardous activity safely decrease as the number of repetitions increase."

WHAT CAUSES OVERUSE INJURY?

According to James Garrick, overuse injuries are most frequently found among people with prior orthopedic problems, those for whom aerobic dance is their only fitness activity, and those who participate infrequently in aerobic dance. He recommends that, to prevent overuse injuries, aerobic-exercise classes feature a gradual but consistent progression in the activity, education regarding the recognition and treatment of overuse injuries, and an exercise leader who can provide appropriate advice on physical complaints.

What Kind of Injuries Occur?

Most injuries in dance exercise occur in the foot (*plantar fasciitis*, a painful inflammation of the connective tissue in the arch of the foot) and the lower leg (shinsplints; knee injury). Research by William Vetter and colleagues show that other sites of common injury include the lower back and neck.

When Are the More Harmful Exercises Performed?

The two parts of a dance-exercise routine that can pose the most danger are strength-building exercises in the floor-exercise portion and stretching exercises in the warmup period. Floor exercises help tone and shape your muscles (although in reality the aerobic portion is just as important in toning and shaping). Their primary goal is to improve muscular strength and endurance. To improve strength, the muscle must be overloaded. This means that it must progressively work against greater resistance. To enhance endurance, the muscle must repeatedly work against a resistance over an extended period of time. Muscular-strength exercises are used to increase strength and promote muscle growth, while muscular-endurance exercises are designed to tone and shape the muscles.

In order to achieve maximum benefit from muscular-strength and endurance exercises, the principle of specificity must be followed. This principle states that in order for a muscle's performance to improve, you must choose exercises for that specific muscle. So, if your goal is to improve your legs, you should select exercises that focus on the legs. Remember, however, performing exercises that focus on the legs will not necessarily result in a loss of fat in the legs. Aerobic exercise and modifications in food intake are the most efficient ways to reduce fat.

The warmup portion of an exercise session is designed to prepare your body for the upcoming vigorous exercise portion of your program. Stretching exercises are normally included as part of the warmup. However, they are used most effectively for increasing flexibility when included in the cool-down portion of the program when the muscle and connective tissue are their warmest. Stretching exercises are included in Chapters 4 through 11.

STAY TUNED

The following chapters analyze common exercises for the neck, shoulder, lower back/abdominals, hip, knee, ankle, and foot. Exercises that place each region at risk are highlighted as are safer alternatives. In addition, a chapter on overuse injury and prevention is included. Exercise should not hurt. The old adage "no pain, no gain" is just flat untrue! Marjorie Albohm warns us that "any exercise that consistently causes discomfort or pain should be eliminated or modified."

FOUR

GET YOUR MOTOR RUNNING

Warming-up

An often ignored but vital component of any exercise session is the warmup. It's tempting to cheat on the warmup portion of your exercise program. You may not feel that you are doing anything productive by including a warmup in your exercise regimen, or you may feel that you don't have time to include a warmup. In dance-exercise classes, there will be people who consistently arrive after the warmup has been completed. This can be very dangerous; your body needs to be prepared for exercise. A body that has been properly warmed-up is capable of performing at a higher level than one that is not.

The warmup period is designed to get your motor running by increasing blood flow to the working muscles, increasing body temperature, and loosening up the muscles for activity. In addition, Barbara Brehm states that the warmup allows your body to increase its production of the hormones responsible for the regulation of energy production. Blood flow to the muscles must increase in order for them to function efficiently and to utilize fat as a fuel source. The oxygen carried in the blood allows you to exercise for a longer time with less fatigue. Increased blood flow to the working muscles also aids in heat dissipation. All of these factors help to decrease your risk of injury.

As you exercise, you also produce heat as a byproduct of the many chemical reactions that occur in your body when you move. These chemical reactions are vital to the proper functioning of your metabolic pathways (energy-transferring pathways). A good warmup will allow you to begin gradually the process of heat production and dissipation. Because a warmer muscle is a more flexible muscle, the warmup aids in loosening up your muscles. The connective tissue that runs in series (is interweaved throughout) and parallel to (alongside) the muscle fibers is similar to elastic. Like elastic, it becomes more pliable when heated, allowing you to move through a full range of motion with less risk of injury.

WHAT SHOULD I DO FOR A WARMUP?

The warmup section of a workout should be composed of low-intensity exercise that is specific (similar) to the exercise that is to follow, and general static (nonbouncing) stretching in which a range of motion is performed. Specificity of training means that, to obtain specific benefits, you must work specific muscles. By utilizing the muscles that will be used more forcefully later, you prepare them for the further demands of exercise, reducing the risk of injury. By also including general flexibility exercises, you ensure that all the muscles that are used in stabilization and as secondary movers are properly prepared.

Low-intensity static (nonbouncing) flexibility exercises should be performed after each muscle has been warmed up through low-intensity movement. A position that puts the muscle on stretch should be assumed; this means placing your body in a position in which the muscle is taken to the longest point in its range of motion and then holding that position. A slight stretching sensation should be felt. Pain, however, should not occur. If the muscle is forced into a position that is stretched too far, it will naturally contract (the *stretch* or *myotatic reflex*) thereby increasing your risk of injury.

The stretching activities included in a warmup are not designed for improvements in long-term flexibility. Their purpose is to prepare the muscles for activity. Long-term flexibility improvement will occur most dramatically in the cool-down portion of an exercise session when the muscle is most pliable. A muscle is warmest after the cardiovascular portion of an exercise session; it is at this time that maximum improvement in flexibility will occur.

SHOULD I ALWAYS AVOID BOUNCING WHEN STRETCHING?

Generally, bouncing stretches should be avoided. However, in some instances, ballistic (bouncing) activities are included in the exercise portion of a workout. Daniel Arnheim defines these ballistic movements as rebounding movements employing an alternate contraction of opposing muscles or groups of muscles. Many exercise professionals feel that ballistic stretching is too dangerous for the recreational exerciser. However, since many activities involve ballistic movement, it can be argued that ballistic stretching has its place in your warmup. It is important to remember that, although ballistic stretching is not a preferred method of warming-up, it can be performed safely if your muscles are fit and properly warmed. For reasons of safety, ballistic stretching should never be the initial form of stretching employed when the muscles are cold.

HOW LONG SHOULD I SPEND WARMING UP?

Your warmup should last a minimum of eight to fifteen minutes. Select exercises that work the muscles that are to be the prime movers in your exercise session. The longer a muscle is placed on stretch, the more flexible it becomes. However, due to time considerations in your exercise session, it is necessary to limit the time each muscle is placed under stretch. A minimum of eight to twelve seconds of stretch for each muscle group to be exercised, performed one to three times, is recommended.

Ruth Lindsey and Charles Corbin remind us to be extremely careful when using stretching exercises in which the body weight, another person, or an object is used to forcefully stretch the muscle. This may cause the muscle to undergo a stretch reflex (myotatic reflex). In a stretch reflex, the muscle that is forcefully stretched elicits a reflex that causes it to contract. If this occurs, the muscle is at an increased risk of tearing. At the same time, this reflex decreases the benefits associated with stretching.

FIVE

IF A LITTLE IS GOOD, MORE MUST BE BETTER

Overuse Syndrome

WHAT IS OVERUSE SYNDROME?

Overuse syndrome refers to the development of pain or injury as the result of too much exercise. Overuse injury is typically related to performing too much too soon, exercising too many days per week, or doing too many repetitions of an activity. Over time, the repetitive nature of an activity may result in long-term damage, particularly if the activity is performed incorrectly. Overuse, or overtraining, plays a significant role in the development of most dance injuries.

WHAT DOES IT FEEL LIKE WHEN I OVERTRAIN?

There are many symptoms associated with overuse syndrome. You may find that you are unable to perform with the same intensity that you normally have, and the quality of your performance may diminish. Cindy Nayer describes overuse symptoms including lethargy, loss of appetite, sudden weight drop, nausea, swelling of the lymph glands, pain in the joints, tendons, or ligaments before or after exercise, or pain that disappears as the exerciser begins warming-up and heat reaches the affected area. Other symptoms may include swelling of a particular area, an increase in the number of colds or other illnesses that you get, or a lingering tingling or numbness in an extremity.

WHAT CAUSES OVERUSE SYNDROME?

Overuse syndrome is related to many different factors. Lyle Micheli describes seven of these factors: training, muscle-tendon imbalance, anatomic malalignment, footwear, surface, growth, and other diseased states.

Training: Change in Frequency and Intensity

A change in training habits or a sudden increase in either the intensity (how hard) or the duration (how long) of exercise may predispose you to overuse syndrome. Richard Norris reports that when professional dancers and dance students abruptly changed the intensity or duration of training, they had the highest rate of injury. This same concept holds true for beginners. Your body requires time to adapt to physical stress, to repair damaged tissue, and to build new tissue. In addition, the body requires rest to restore energy in the muscles. When you reduce this recovery time, your body cannot rebuild muscle tissue and will be more susceptible to stress-related injury.

Muscle-Tendon Imbalance

Muscle-tendon imbalance occurs when the muscle is too weak or too inflexible to support an activity. Additionally, a muscle may be stronger than the supporting tendon, putting the tendon at a greater risk of rupturing. A balanced training regimen including symmetrical strength training (working all muscles evenly) and specific stretching exercises can help to guard against this condition. For example, working on the calf muscles only while ignoring the muscles of the front part of the leg (*anterior tibialis*) may result in shin pain. Warming-up and cooling-down are also critical in preventing acute (sudden) onset of this problem.

Anatomic Malalignment

Improper body positioning and individual variations in body build can cause anatomic malalignment. In addition, poor muscular development or muscular imbalance may also contribute to this condition. In other words, what you have just doesn't fit together properly. Anatomic malalignment usually takes one of two forms. It can be functional, meaning that it is related to a muscle's weakness or inflexibility, or it can be structural, meaning that it is related to abnormal bone formation.

This condition, once it makes itself known, should be treated first by identifying the causative factors, then working to reduce their influence. For instance, if a strength imbalance is found to be the cause, a strength and conditioning program may alleviate the symptoms. If an anatomical deviation exists due to bone structure, supporting devices such as orthotics may be prescribed. If malalignment problems are suspected, check with your physician for proper treatment.

Footwear

As we stated in Chapter 2, proper footwear is a must. When you land in an active exercise, your feet must absorb forces in excess of three times your body weight. To handle these forces, you should select shoes that provide enough traction to prevent slippage and enough stability to support the muscles of your feet and lower legs. Good shoes will be light enough to allow mobility and yet durable enough to provide cushioning for shock absorption.

Surface

As discussed in Chapter 2, good surfaces will decrease the impact forces associated with dance exercise. The surface should minimize slippage and provide a firm yet shock-absorbing exercise area. Spring-mounted wooden floors, commonly found in many gymnasiums and dance studios, are universally recognized as the best surface for dance-exercise classes.

Growth

As a young individual ages, rapid growth occurs, which may result in muscle imbalance and a decreased ability of the muscles to handle the stress associated with exercise. It is generally agreed that young individuals are quite capable of vigorous exercise. However, it is important to remember to modify exercise procedures for younger exercisers to fit their rapidly changing bodies (see Chapter 2).

Other Associated Disease States

When other associated disease states exist, you should not exercise. For instance, when an infection occurs, additional stress is placed upon the body. Exercising will endanger an already weakened body. It is better to allow the disease process to run its course before exercising. Otherwise, you may prolong your illness.

SUMMARY

Overuse injuries may take on a variety of symptoms. According to Richard Norris, "The most common injuries are from overuse, or in medical terms, repetitive microtrauma rather than a single gross incident of macrotrauma. The result may take the form of tendonitis, stress fractures in the lower extremities, or pain about the kneecap." Changes in technique can also bring about similar results. Most overuse injury takes one of two forms. Accumulated microtrauma (minor injuries) caused by repetitive motion can result in inflammation, which may cause *bursa* (the liquid-filled sacks that cushion the joints) and tendon pain. Or the accumulated microtrauma, if not given enough time to heal, can lead to tendon ruptures, stress fractures, and *plantar fasciitis* (inflammation of the muscle at the base of the foot).

Overuse injury is the factor most associated with dance-exercise injury, and is usually caused by poor technique and exercise practices. It can be prevented by following the recommended guidelines for exercise participation, being careful of body alignment, and by learning about exercises that increase your risk of injury.

SIX

A REAL PAIN IN THE NECK

Neck Exercises

The neck is a vital part of the human body, supporting the head and protecting the spinal column. Because of its structure, the neck region is easily injured. There are numerous exercises that can put the neck at risk. Ellen Kreighbaum states that "the cervical vertebrae can be injured when body weight is placed on the neck area, and the thoracic area can be injured when the thoracic vertebrae are forced into an extreme forward-bending posture." Although any neck injury should be avoided, the cervical spine (neck vertebrae) is the primary area of concern. The spinal column protects the nerves that transmit impulses to and from the brain. Damage to this portion of the spine could lead to severe paralysis or death.

WHAT EXERCISES PUT THE NECK AT RISK?

Neck hyperflexion (bending the head too far forward) and neck hyperextension (bending the head too far backward) are the two major types of exercise that put the neck at risk. Protection of the neck is of paramount importance in any exercise situation, because many exercises are performed that cause hyperflexion and hyperextension. These positions weaken the support of the head by transferring support primarily to the cervical spine. Other injuries to the neck will most likely occur in ballistic (rapid movement) activities. Because the head is relatively massive and heavy, ballistic movement can cause very large torque (rotary force) at the neck. This torque must be supported by the musculature of the neck and the cervical vertebrae. If the torque is too large or the muscle too weak, injury to the vertebrae may occur. A pinching together on one side of the spine produces tremendous forces on the opposite side that may lead to disc herniation (a ballooning of the disc membrane) or rupturing (a break in the membrane).

AVOID OR MODIFY THESE EXERCISES

Neck Hyperflexion

Many exercises aggravate pre-existing conditions. Charles Corbin and Ruth Lindsey estimate that 80 percent of the population have forward head position (the head leans forward like a turtle's) and kyphosis (rounding of the upper back). They warn that "exercises that tend to promote or aggravate these conditions by further stretching already elongated muscles and ligaments should be avoided." In general, any exercise that places abnormally high stress on the cervical spine should be avoided. The following exercises put the neck into potentially dangerous positions of hyperflexion (bending too far forward).

1. Plough

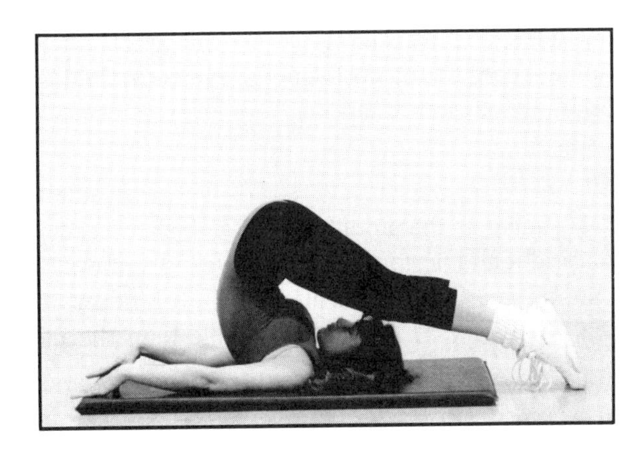

The plough is a yoga exercise that is designed to stretch the musculature of the lower back. In this position, however, the entire weight of the body must be supported by the neck and shoulders. The neck is in a vulnerable position, which is compounded by the application of huge compressive forces at the anterior (front) portion of the cervical spine. Researchers generally agree that this places stress on the posterior (rear) portion of the vertebrae.

2. *Plough shear*

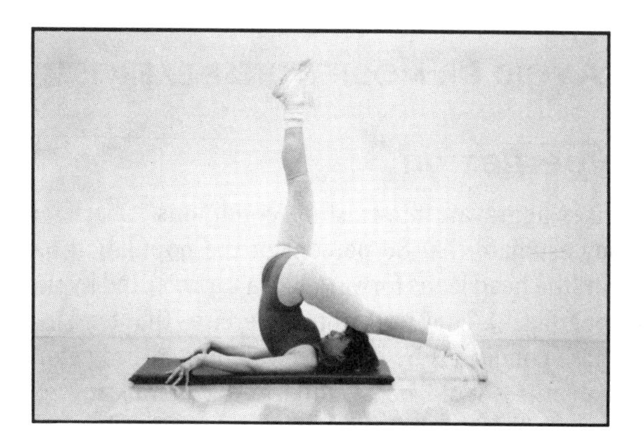

This exercise is similar to the plough, with the exception that only one leg is brought to the floor over the head while the other is held in a vertical position, and, according to Charles Corbin and Ruth Lindsey, it has similar risks. It can be even more dangerous than the plough because your body is in a less stable position; there is one less contact point with the floor, thus reducing the base of support and your ability to maintain your balance.

3. *Vertical cycling*

This position is similar to the plough and plough shear, except that both legs are held upright and perform a vertical cycling motion. According to both Karen Smith, and Charles Corbin and Ruth Lindsey, it shares the same potential for injury. It is even less stable than the plough shear

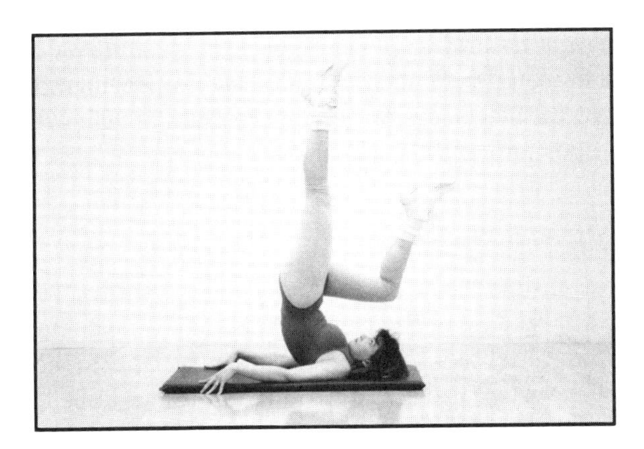

because two contact points with the floor have been removed, increasing the likelihood that you will lose your balance. By removing these two contact points from the base of support, there is also a greater shift in ground-reaction force (support force) to the shoulders and spine that must now support the entire body weight. The cycling movement of the legs adds an undesirable ballistic component to the stretch.

4. Sit-up with hands behind the head

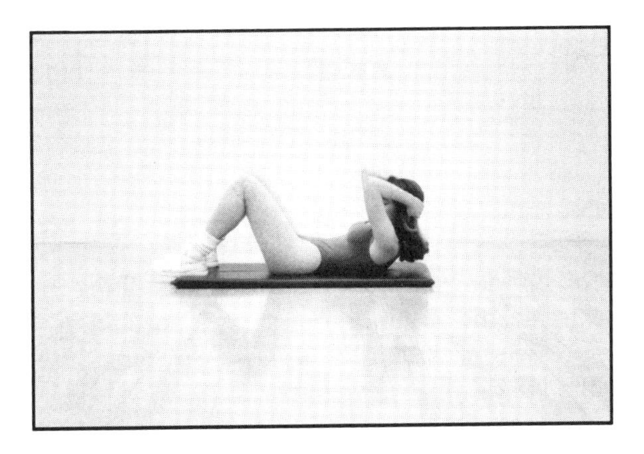

A different type of exercise that endangers the neck is the sit-up with hands clasped behind the head. When you clasp your hands behind your head, you have a natural tendency to pull the head forward, especially when you're tired. Helen Timmermans and Malissa Martin report that this application of torque places large compressive forces on the anterior aspect (front portion) of the cervical spine.

Neck Hyperextension

Neck hyperextension occurs when your head is bent too far backward, resulting in a spreading of the front portion and a pinching of the rear portion of the vertebrae. These exercises may lead to herniation or rupture of the vertebral discs. According to Adele Lubell, the neural foramen (the area through which the nerve roots pass) may narrow due to neck hyperextension, especially if you suffer from degenerative disc disease.

1. Neck hyperextension by looking up

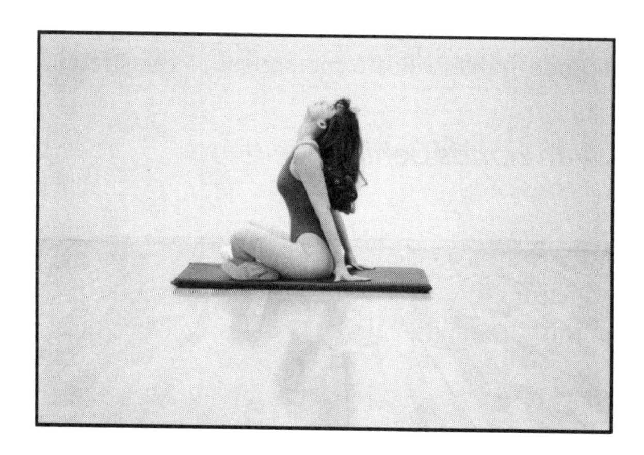

When you look up with your neck hyperextended, tilting the head backward to its extreme, the posterior aspect (back portion) of your cervical spine is compressed. According to many researchers, this activity also compresses the arteries that serve the brain.

2. Head circling

Circling your head backward hyperextends the neck. The ballistic quality of the movement further aggravates the problem caused by Exercise 1. According to Charles Corbin and Ruth Lindsey, "Tipping the head backward during any exercise, such as is done in neck circling, can pinch arteries and nerves at the base of the skull and result in dizziness or myofascial trigger points. Therefore, backward tilting of the head is not recommended for many people." Myofascial trigger points are areas of pain brought on by a muscle remaining in a state of contraction and irritating a nerve.

3. Bridging

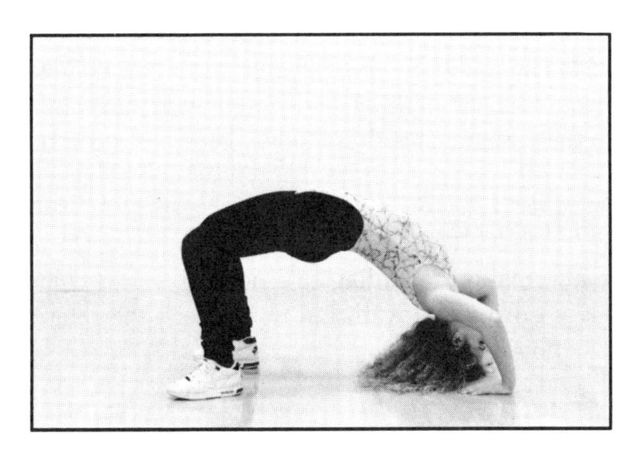

Adele Lubell points out that neck bridging (arching backward to balance on the feet, hands, and head), as frequently performed by wrestlers, hyperextends the neck. The dangers of neck hyperextension are heightened further by the movement (frequently neck circling) that is commonly performed by the exerciser. This causes similar problems as in head circling, with the additional weight of the body making it even more dangerous.

Guidelines for Safe and Effective Neck Exercises

The neck is composed of several muscle groups that you may exercise safely if you know what you are doing. These major muscle groups include the *sternocleidomastoids* (the large muscles that you can easily see when you turn your head to the side) and the *trapezius* (the triangular-shaped muscle found at the base of the neck). Research shows that there are no problems with neck exercises when they are performed through the normal range of motion and performed slowly and under control.

There are several points to consider for protecting the neck. The major dangers come from overloading the neck in positions in which the musculature cannot handle the weight; neck hyperflexion is one such position. The neck may have an additional load, such as the weight of the body, placed on it when performing the plough, placing it at unusual risk. Therefore, neck flexion should only be performed without any additional load applied to the cervical spine.

The other position of concern is neck hyperextension. Extension of the neck is safe and necessary; however, hyperextension should be avoided. The head should not be tilted backward to its extreme, especially when a load is applied. The additional load in this condition may come from a partner or from the momentum associated with movement. Ballistic (bouncing) activity aggravates these movements and position.

Safe Alternatives

Much of our information regarding safe neck exercises comes from the work of Charles Corbin and Ruth Lindsey. Check the reference list for further information on this topic.

1. Ear to shoulder

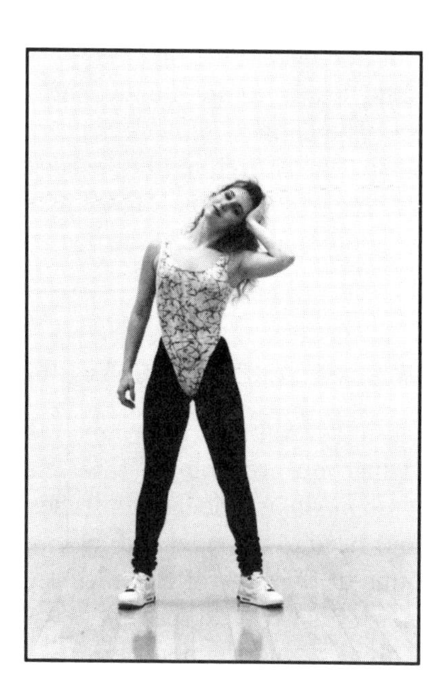

Slowly drop your left ear to the left shoulder. Charles Corbin and Ruth

Lindsey suggest that you apply resistance with your hand while moving the ear toward your shoulder. The movement should be slow and controlled. Hold this position for several seconds, then release to a neutral position. Repeat the movement in the opposite direction. It is important to remember that both sides should be exercised equally.

2. Neck rotation

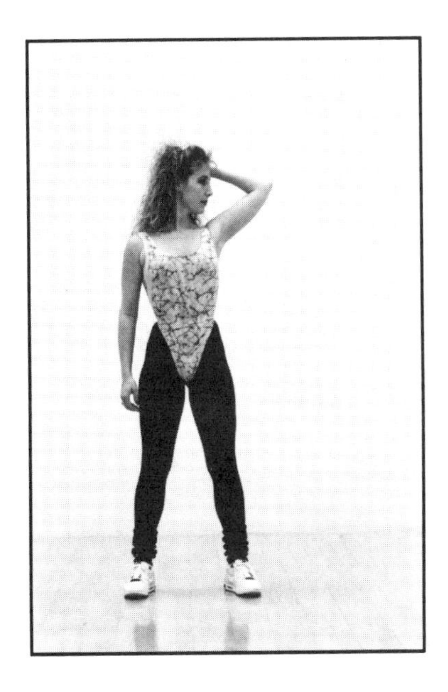

Slowly turn your head to the left, while applying resistance with your hand to the left side of your head. Then, remove your hand and immediately turn your head in the opposite direction, applying resistance with your right hand. In this exercise, the head rotates right and left; there is no upward or downward tilting of the head. This exercise will develop strength in the neck musculature without risking damage to the vertebrae.

3. Neck stretch

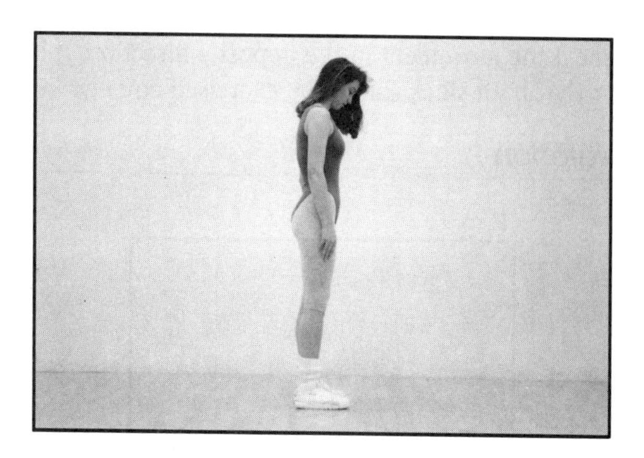

Roll your head slowly in a half-circle from one side, forward, to the opposite side. You should not make a full circle by tipping the head back.

4. Neck flexion exercise

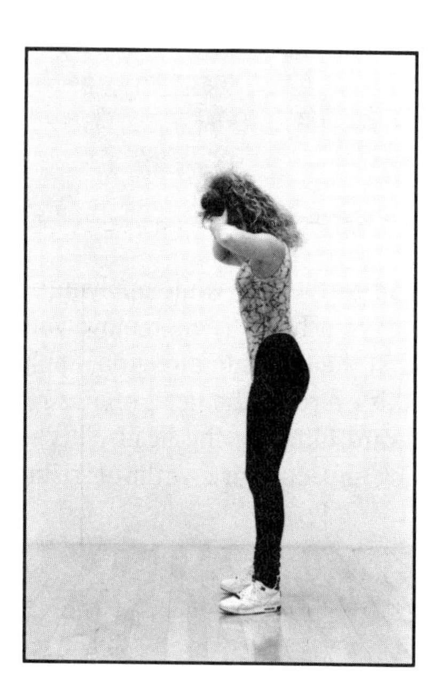

Place both hands on your forehead to provide resistance while you try to move your head forward into flexion. Avoid hyperflexion.

5. Isometric neck pull

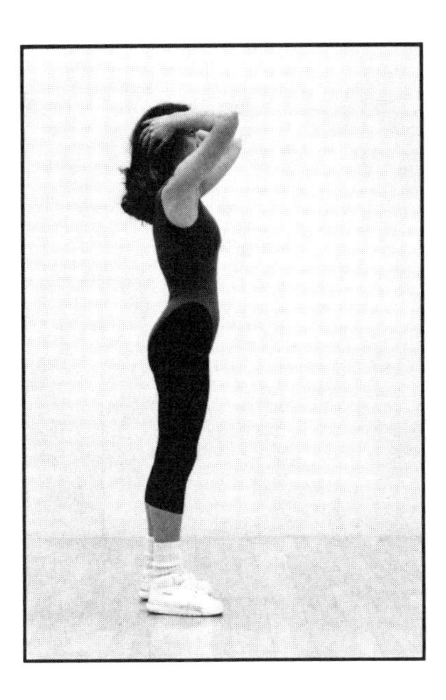

Interlock your fingers behind your head with your elbows pointing forward. Pull your head forward with your hands, resisting the pull by pushing backward with your head. Don't pull your neck into hyperflexion.

6. Neck extension exercise

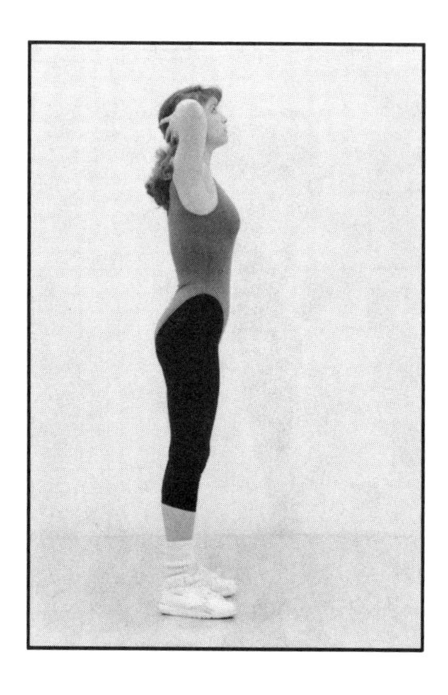

Place both hands at the back of your head to provide resistance while you try to move your head into extension (backward). Avoid hyperextending your neck.

7. Sit-up with hands on shoulders

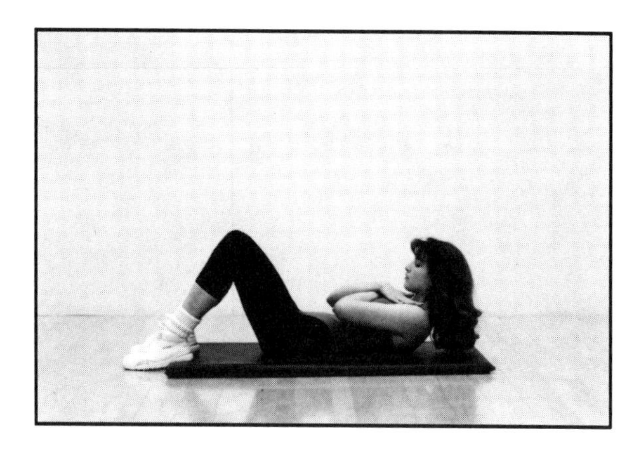

Sit-ups are important for building optimal abdominal strength and endurance. By placing your hands on your shoulders, you eliminate the tendency to pull on your neck when your abdominal muscles become fatigued, which allows you to safely exercise the abdominals without risking injury to the neck. If you need to support your head when performing a sit-up, place your hands at the side of your head by the ears.

SUMMARY

The neck is an extremely vulnerable area and must be protected during exercise. Exercises that develop the neck musculature can aid in this protection, without putting the neck at risk. By exercising the neck regularly and avoiding positions of hyperextension and hyperflexion, especially with an external load applied, the neck musculature will get stronger, and you will protect the cervical vertebrae from injury.

SEVEN

KEEP YOUR SHOULDER TO THE WHEEL

Shoulder Exercises

The shoulder is composed of the insertion of the upper arm (*humerus*) into the socket formed by the collar bone (*clavicle*) and the shoulder blade (*scapula*) and is supported by a series of muscles, tendons, and ligaments. The most common problems associated with the shoulder are a partial "popping out" (subluxation) or a complete dislocation of the *humerus*. Typically, these injuries are the result of an imbalance of force applied to the region and occur most frequently in a collision or during rapid movement activities.

You can increase the stability of this joint by strengthening its musculature. Many exercisers work the musculature of this region, but fail to do so symmetrically. Typically, the muscles that cause forward rotation of the shoulder are exercised while the muscles that cause backward rotation are ignored. This imbalance can result in a form of overuse injury called shoulder-impingement syndrome (a pinching of the nerve that runs through the shoulder region), a rounding of the shoulders (kyphosis), or increased risk of subluxation and dislocation.

AVOID OR MODIFY THESE EXERCISES

There are three areas of concern when exercising the shoulder region. The first is muscular imbalance, which we have already discussed. According to Charles Corbin and Ruth Lindsey, "Exercises that cause muscle imbalance should be avoided. Frequently one set of muscles is overdeveloped while opposing muscles are neglected. This causes misalignment of the body." Richard Norris warns that dancing does not promote equal development of all muscle groups, and further suggests that muscle-tendon imbalance can lead to abnormal forces across the shoulder joint and ultimately can cause injury.

The second area of concern involves very large, rapid arm-rotation movements (particularly arm circles) with the palms facing down. Charles Corbin and Ruth Lindsey explain that this activity may lead to shoulder injury. A third potential problem occurs when shoulder exercises involve keeping the arms above shoulder level for extended periods of time.

1. Forward-only motions

Exercises that emphasize movement in only one direction may lead to muscular imbalance, for example focusing only on push-ups and bench pressing. Charles Corbin and Ruth Lindsey point out that "a common example is the overuse of exercises to strengthen the pectorals while neglecting the *rhomboid* and *trapezius* muscles between the shoulder blades. This results in round shoulders."

2. Arms above shoulder level

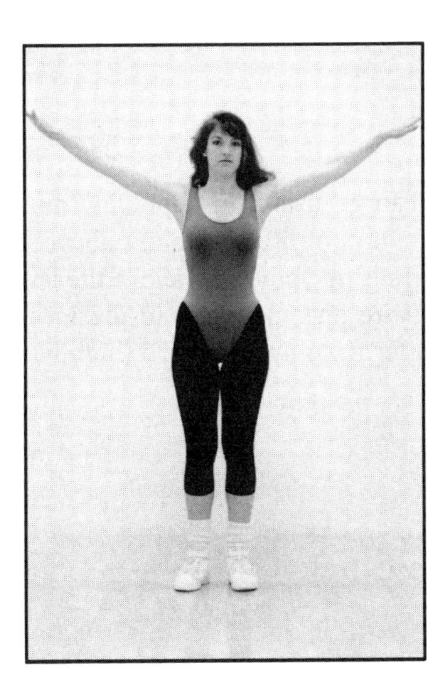

Prolonged exercising while holding your arms above shoulder level (such as is done when performing shoulder circles) can lead to shoulder strain and result in an excessive rise in your blood pressure. According to Ken

Alan, these exercises can also result in excessive tension in the *trapezius* muscles. Karen Clippinger-Robertson suggests that excessive overhead arm movements with poor mechanics can lead to shoulder-impingement syndrome.

3. *Holding hand weights above the heart*

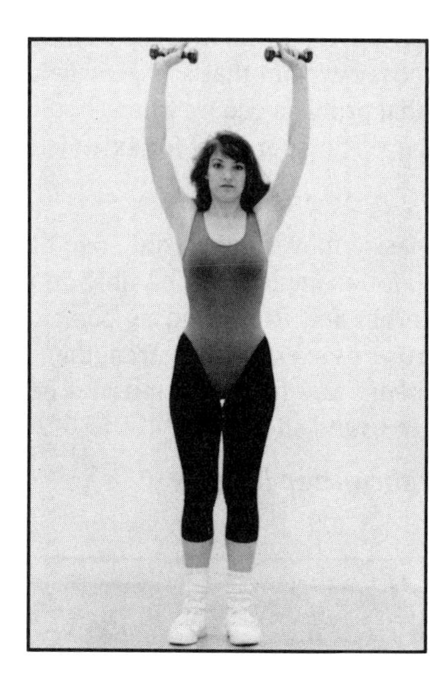

Hand-held weights can be useful in improving muscular strength and endurance. However, do not lift the weight above your heart for more than a few seconds. Raising your arms above the level of your heart will increase blood pressure and may lead to dizziness. This can be very dangerous if you suffer from hypertension (high blood pressure).

4. *Arm circles with the palm facing down*

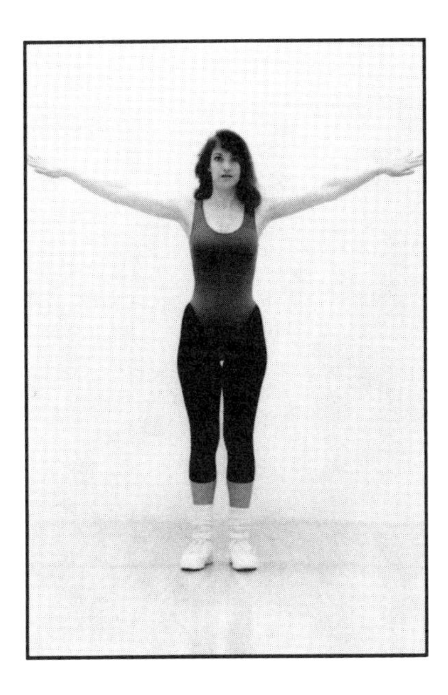

Performing repetitive arm circles with the palms of the hands facing down increases the risk for rotator cuff injuries. According to Ruth Lindsey and Charles Corbin, you are usually unaware of the wear and tear associated with this movement until, over time, the friction wears down the tendon and/or the tuberosity of the *humerus* resulting in tendonitis, bursitis, and arthritis (inflammation of the tendon, *bursa,* and joint, respectively).

Guidelines for Safe and Effective Shoulder Exercises

Exercising the musculature of the shoulder region is important; however, balanced exercising is a must. Exercises that work all of the muscles of the shoulder should be included in your fitness program. Note that your arms should always be kept lower than your shoulders when you perform arm-circling exercises. If your arms are taken above shoulder level in any exercise, they should remain raised only for a brief period of time. Arm rotations should only be performed with the palms turned up. A rhythmical exercise pattern (arms and/or shoulders up and down for short periods of time) is less likely to cause dangerous increases in blood pressure.

Safe Alternatives

1. Pectoral stretch

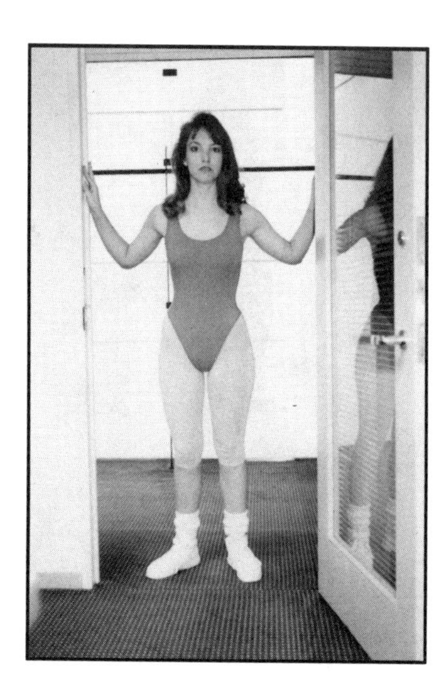

Stand in a doorway with your hands positioned against the doorframe and lean forward, keeping the body in a straight line from the feet to the head. You should feel the stretch across the chest and shoulders, the pectoral region.

2. Wand exercise

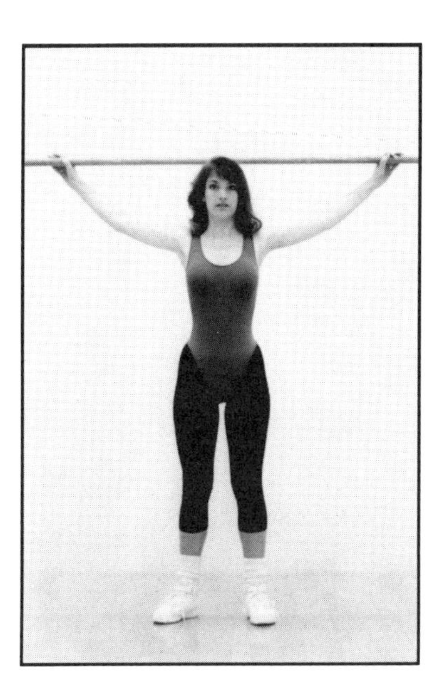

Holding a wand or broomstick horizontally in front of your body, approximately waist-high, slowly lift the wand over your head to your back. Keep your arms straight and do not release your grip while moving the wand. According to Charles Corbin and Ruth Lindsey, the stretch should be felt primarily throughout the shoulder region and possibly in the arms.

3. Arms across chest

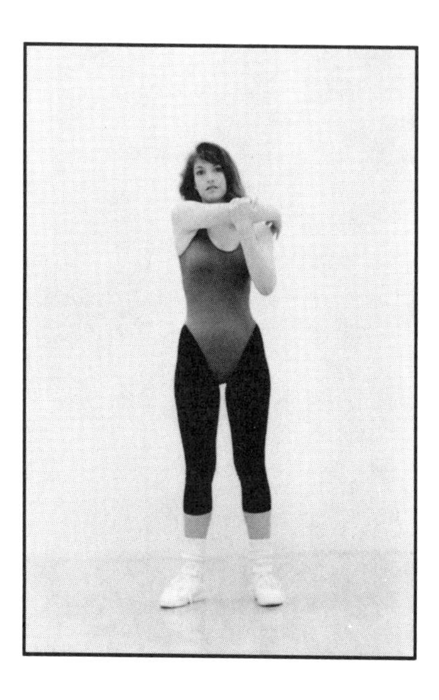

Bring your left arm across your chest at shoulder level. Hold this position for ten seconds. Use your right arm to apply pressure to increase the stretch. This pressure should be applied gradually above the elbow joint on the upper arm. Repeat with your other arm.

4. Back scratch

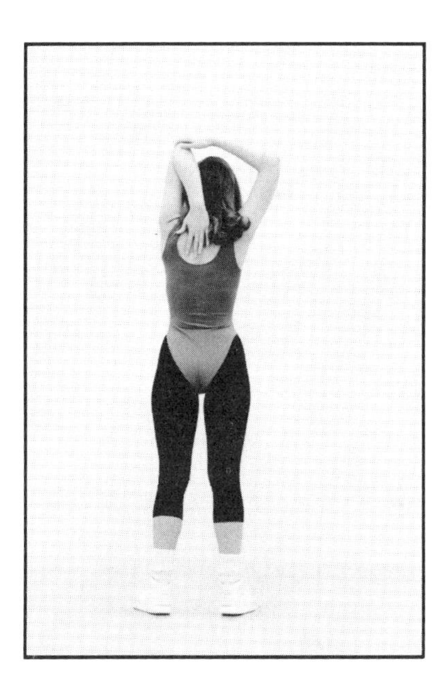

Raise your left arm with your elbow pointing toward the ceiling and your hand reaching back and down to "scratch your back." Hold this position while applying light pressure below your left elbow with your right hand. Repeat the exercise with your other arm. Be aware of a tendency to arch the lower back as the arms are taken overhead. Protect your back by keeping your abdominals tight and your pelvis tucked in.

Suggested Shoulder-Strengthening Exercises

1. Bench pressing

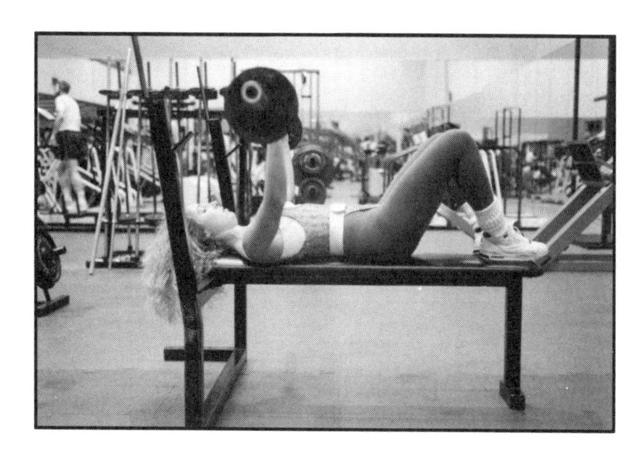

This exercise will improve the strength of the anterior head (front portion) of the *deltoids* (shoulder muscle) as well as the *pectoralis* (chest muscles) and *triceps* (muscles of the back of the upper arm). Your lower back should not be arched when you are bench pressing, and you should maintain a steady breathing pattern and constant muscle tension.

2. Rowing

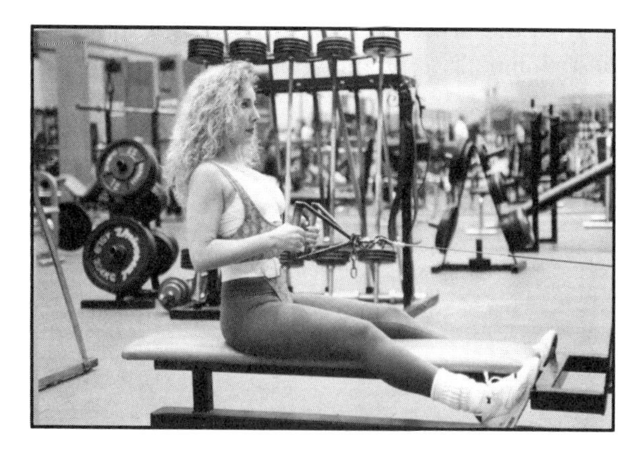

This exercise will develop the posterior head of the *deltoids* (shoulder) as well as the *biceps* (muscles located on the front of the upper arm) and *latissimus dorsi* (V-shaped muscle in the upper back). Make sure that you don't arch your lower back when moving against the resistance of the rowing machine.

SUMMARY

The key to shoulder stability is properly developed shoulder strength. To achieve this goal, each of the shoulders' muscle groups must be symmetrically developed. While developing shoulder strength, you should avoid isometric (nonmoving) exercises that involve holding your arms overhead, because they can cause a dangerous increase in your blood pressure.

EIGHT

OH MY ACHING BACK!

Back Exercises

The lower back is one of the most often injured areas of the body. According to Ellen Kelly, lower back injuries are seldom related to one simple traumatic event, but are usually the result of repeated minor injury or overuse.

Proper lower-back fitness is critical in preventing lower-back pain. Exercises that injure the lower back often are not those specifically designed to work on the back. Rather, the lower back is typically injured when you are trying to exercise another part of the body.

HOW COMMON IS LOWER-BACK PAIN?

Charles Corbin and Ruth Lindsey point out that lower-back pain is the number one medical complaint in the United States. Statistics show that 80 to 85 percent of all back pain is the result of poor muscle fitness, including poor flexibility, and a lack of strength and muscle endurance. Furthermore, William Stone reports that 80 percent of American adults will experience back pain at some time in their lives. Any exercise program should include preventative and rehabilitative care of the lower back.

WHICH MUSCLES ARE INVOLVED?

The key muscle groups that contribute to lower-back fitness are the hamstrings (back of the thigh), the abdominals (stomach), the hip flexors, and the back extensors. These muscles must be properly exercised to guard against back pain. A balanced exercise program for the muscles of the lower back is critical. According to Ellen Kreighbaum, "The lumbar vertebrae, which are the largest vertebrae in the back, can be easily injured during trunk-strengthening exercises, particularly if the abdominals are weak." Weak abdominal muscles cause you to arch the lower back, leading to lower-back pain.

AVOID OR MODIFY THESE EXERCISES

As with many of the other joints, hyperflexion (too much flexion) and hyperextension (too much extension) may put the lower back at risk. Carol Goodman notes that repetitive flexion exercises can cause gradual, long-term changes in the lower back because of the hinge action of the spine at this point. Ellen Kelly warns that a forward slippage of the last lumbar vertebrae (second lowest part of the spine) on the *sacrum* (lowest part of the spine) may cause immediate pain and can lead to further injury, including a stress fracture.

Many factors contribute to these problems. Back pain in dancers is usually related to flaws in their dance technique. Ellen Kelly states, "Repetitive use of poor technique and body mechanics generate musculoskeletal imbalance and ultimately leads to injury. The spine will give out at its weakest point, straining muscles, spraining ligaments, and injuring discs. Stress fractures can even result from repetitive impacting on vertebral arches."

Here are some of the most common exercises that cause back injuries and some safer alternatives. When evaluating these exercises, we need to keep in mind their purpose: Do they really achieve what we want, and do we need to perform them in order to meet our exercise objectives?

Back Hyperextension

Exercises that excessively hyperextend (overarch) the spine can lead to osteoarthritis (inflammation of the bones and joints), muscle stiffness, disc degeneration, tendon strains, and osteoporosis (loss of bone).

1. Straight-leg sit-ups

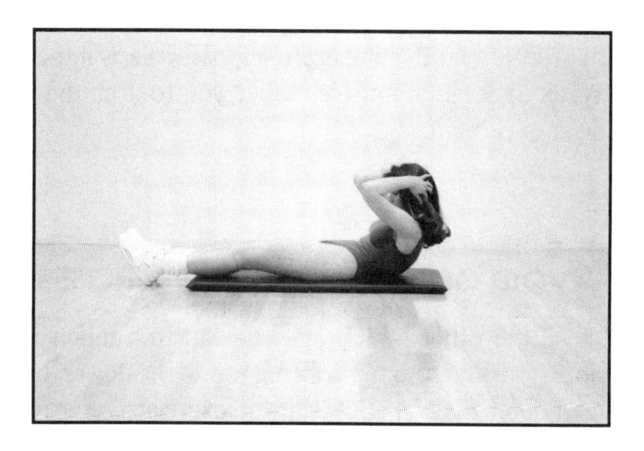

When you perform straight-leg sit-ups, you use the hip flexors (groin muscles) to rise to a sitting position. In addition, Daniel Arnheim reports that your lower back is often hyperextended to assist in the rising motion of the exercise. For this reason, this type of sit-up should be avoided. Keep in mind that straight-leg sit-ups strengthen the hip-flexor muscles primarily, rather than the abdominals. As the hip flexors become stronger, especially without matching strength in the abdominals, there is increased arching in the lower back, contributing to lower-back pain. The hip-flexor muscles are exercised every time you take a step while walking, and, for the average person, these muscles need little (if any) additional strengthening. Generally, they require stretching rather than strengthening.

2. Double leg raises

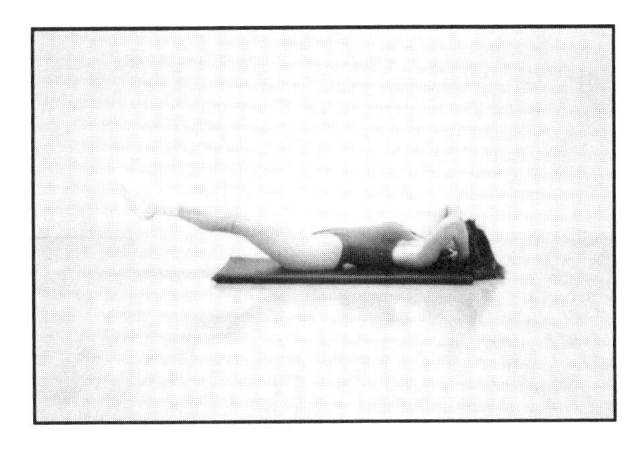

Double leg raises cause a forward tilt of the pelvis resulting in hyperextension of the lower back and strengthening of the hip flexors, particularly if you have weak abdominal muscles. The double leg-lift exercise causes the *iliopsoas* muscle (a groin muscle) to contract, exaggerating the curve of the lower back and contributing to lower-back pain.

3. Donkey kicks

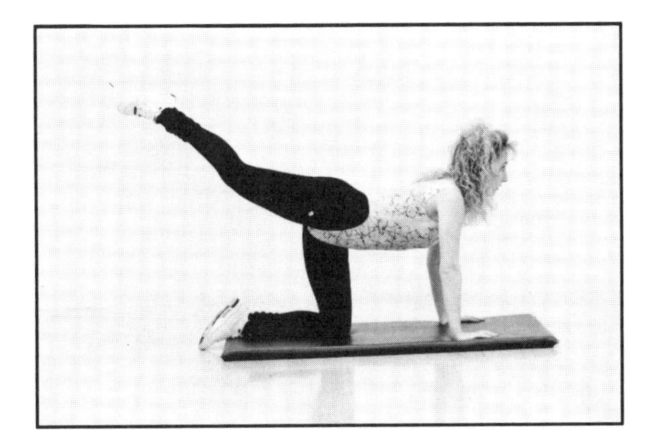

This exercise is performed in an all-fours position on the floor to strengthen the *gluteal* (buttocks) and hamstring muscles. A single-leg raise or knee-to-nose movement with a backward kick are standard movements that are performed from this position. The donkey kick causes hyperextension of the lumbar spine. You are at greatest risk when you try to "work harder" by raising the kicking leg above hip level.

4. Back bends/bridges

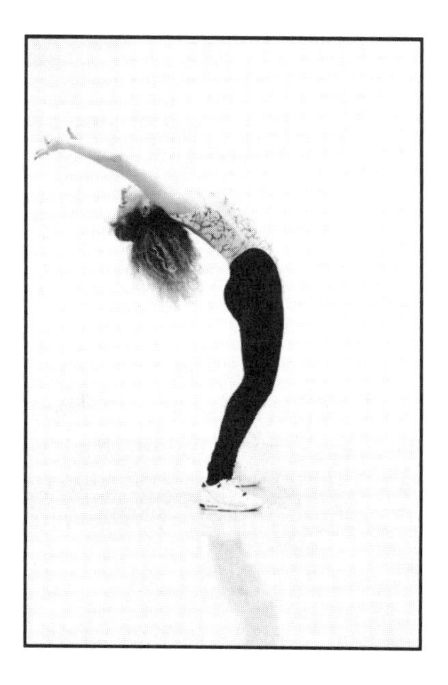

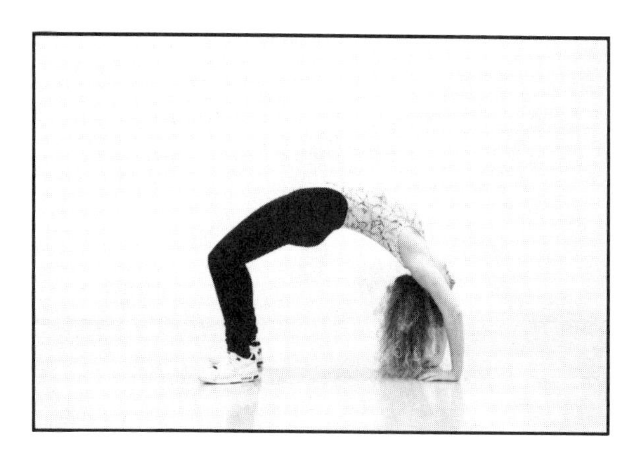

Back bends, particularly when performed in a standing position, may cause lower-back hyperextension. Karen Smith mentions that the bridge position, which adds the stress of supporting the body's weight to this exercise, endangers the lumbar spine (lower back).

5. Trunk rotations

Dynamic (rapidly moving) trunk rotations increase the risk associated with performing back bends. The momentum of the moving body adds significant torque (rotational force) to the stresses placed upon the lumbar region.

6. Cobra

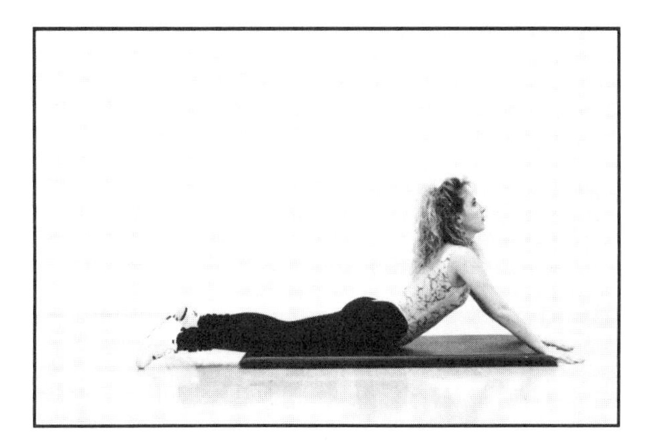

The cobra position is a yoga position designed to stretch the abdominal muscles. This position causes extreme hyperextension of the lumbar spine. It is generally agreed that you should be more concerned with strengthening the abdominal muscles than with stretching them. Safe abdominal stretching can be performed in the supine position with your back pressed flat to the floor and your arms reaching horizontally overhead.

7. Hip extension in prone (face-down-on-floor) position

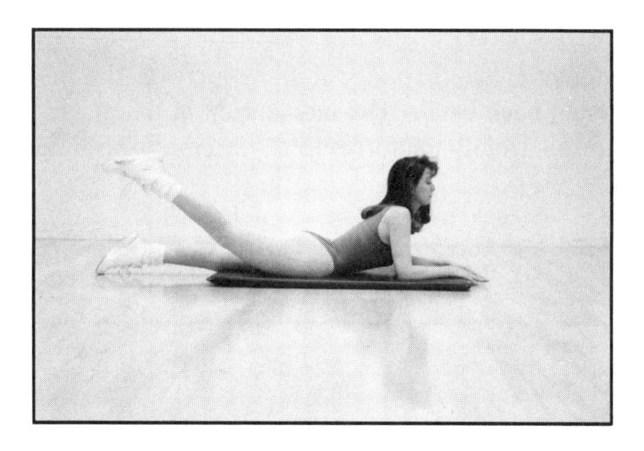

This movement is similar to the donkey kick with the exception that you are prone (lying face down on the floor) instead of on all-fours. As in the donkey kick, raising your leg above your buttocks results in a pelvic tilt that hyperextends the lower back.

8. Prone position, reaching back and grabbing the feet

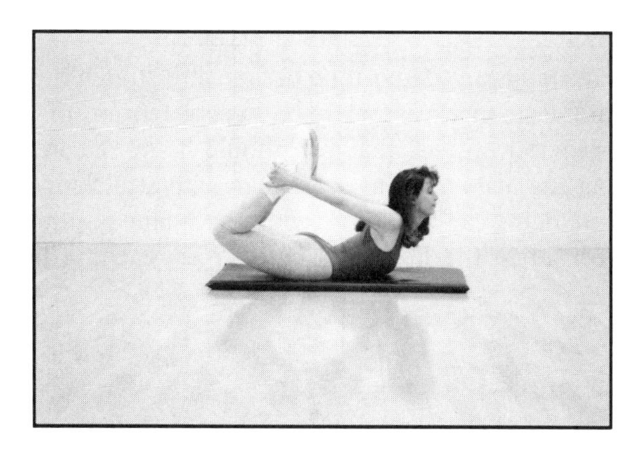

This stretching exercise is designed to improve flexibility in the abdominal and *quadricep* (front of the thigh) regions. Not only is your lower back forced into a position of hyperextension, but your knees are placed in a position of hyperflexion. This may lead to multijoint injury.

9. Sitting on the heels and bending backward to stretch the abdominals

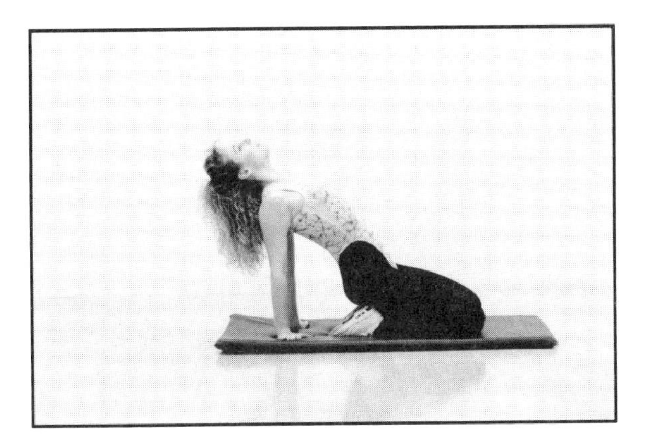

As in Exercise 8, the lower back is hyperextended and the knees are hyperflexed by this movement.

10. Side bends with arms overhead

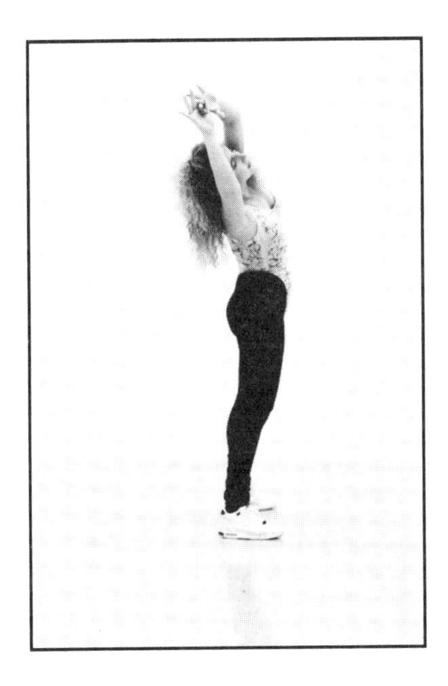

According to Ken Alan, this movement frequently results in forward flexion and rotation of the back, increasing pressure on the lumbar discs.

Additionally, when you lean back and to the side, your lower back is placed in a position of hyperextension, causing unnecessary stress on your lumbar spine. This exercise can be performed safely by eliminating forward or backward rotation and by raising only one arm overhead at a time.

11. Arched back push-ups

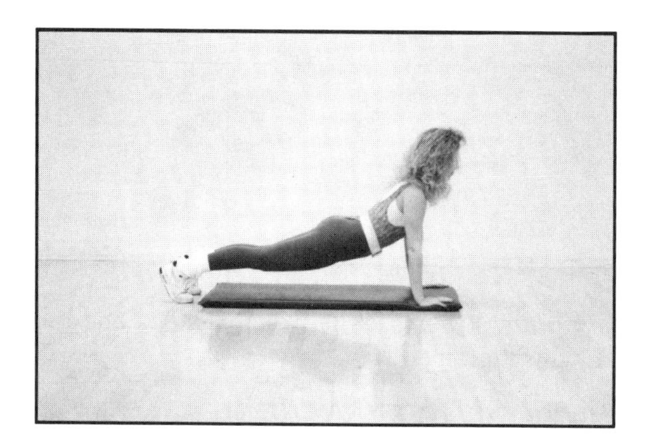

Even the common push-up, if performed incorrectly, can result in injury. When you perform push-ups with an arched back, your lumbar vertebrae may be compressed excessively. You should maintain a normal curve in your back by contracting your abdominal muscles.

12. Leg scissoring

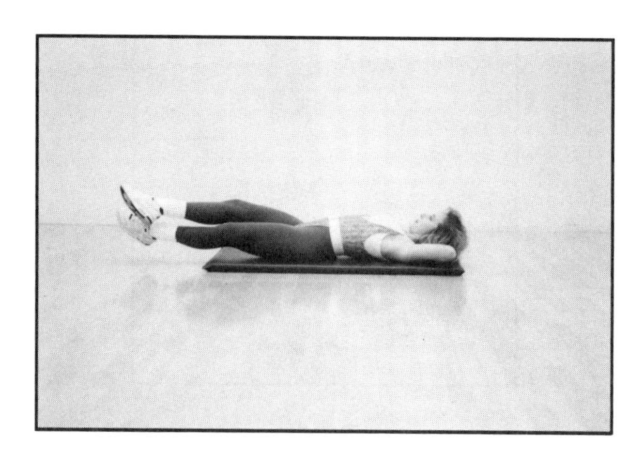

Lie on your back with your heels off the floor, while alternately moving your legs in a side-to-side crossing motion. This exercise is ineffective for strengthening your abdominal muscles because you primarily use your hip flexors to perform it. It is also dangerous because you will inevitably arch your lower back while performing it.

13. Fire hydrants

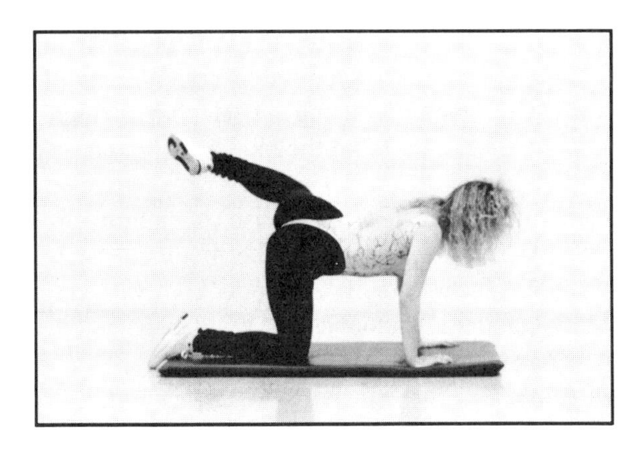

Bend your leg and raise it to your side from an all-fours position. This exercise puts undue strain on the ligaments supporting your hip joint and may result in laxity (looseness) of those ligaments. In addition, if you bring your leg above hip level, hyperextension of your lower back may occur, leading to an increased risk of back injury. You may also strain your hip rotator muscles because they must generate tremendous force to perform this activity.

Back Hyperflexion

Bending too far forward (hyperflexion) may be as risky as arching your back and may predispose you to tension injuries.

1. Forward flexion (touching your toes)

This type of movement (standing and touching your toes) is very controversial. The argument against these exercises, outlined by Paula Besson, is that far too much weight (the whole upper torso) has to be supported by the lower spine. By forcing the lower back to support this extra weight, these exercises may cause traumatic injury to the musculature, discs, or ligaments of the area.

Each part of the spine is made up of bone separated by a disc that contains a gelatinous center surrounded by a rubberlike ring. During flexion of the trunk, the front borders of the intervertebral discs are compressed. This compression forces the gelatinous material backward and stretches the ring. The pressure can be so great that the ring tears, allowing the gelatinous material to leak outward and become trapped against the ligament along the back of the spine.

Overuse injuries may also be caused by this type of activity. By repeatedly bending as far forward as possible, while using the muscles of the lower back to support the weight of the body, the muscles and ligaments in the area may become overstretched. Overstretched ligaments decrease joint stability and increase the risk of joint injury. Additionally, when you perform this exercise, your hamstring muscles are stretched and contracted at the same time, increasing the likelihood that a hamstring tear will occur.

The argument for forward-flexion exercises is that forward flexion is a natural movement. These exercises can be modified if you bend your knees to help support the weight of your upper body with your legs. It has been argued that eliminating a movement that is a part of your daily life may actually increase your risk for injury.

It is our view that flexion and extension are necessary, but that positions of hyperflexion and hyperextension, especially when they include additional loading or bouncing, should be avoided.

2. Windmills

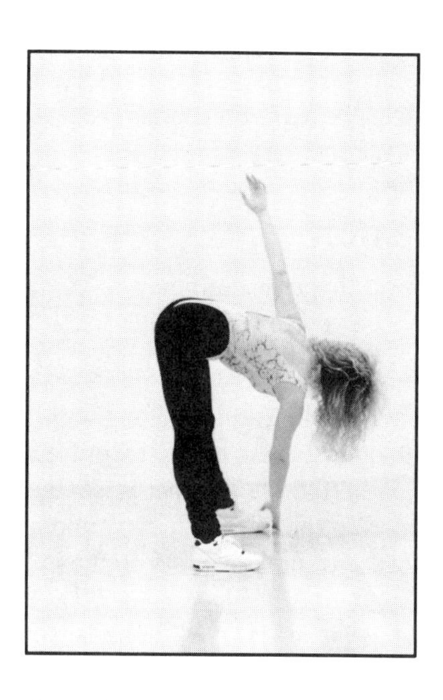

When you perform dynamic movements such as windmills (alternate toe touches), the torque produced from the rotary motion is added to the stress already being applied to your spine by forward flexion. Not only can the downward movement cause hyperflexion of the lumbar spine when you lean forward, but the recovery motion causes hyperextension of the lower spine.

According to Susan Calhoun, the increased pressure in the discs, caused by the forces associated with the down-and-across movements, may tear the rings around the discs, potentially driving fluid inside each disc diagonally backward. If this herniated mass bypasses the longitudinal ligament and comes in direct contact with the nerve root, sciatic nerve pain can occur.

3. *Standing toe touches*

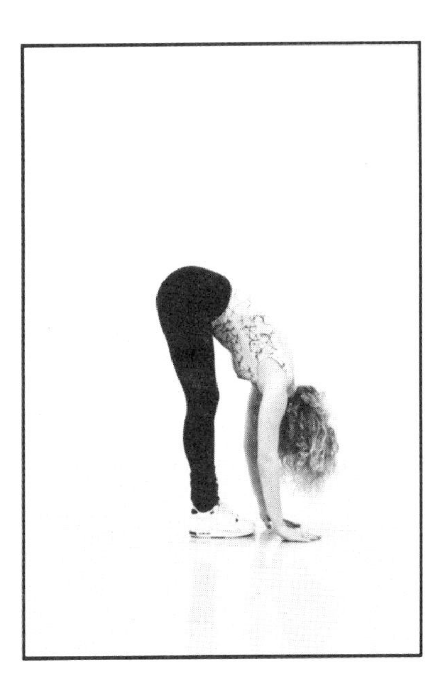

Toe touches are a dynamic exercise in which you alternately reach down and try to touch your toes and then return to an upright position. This exercise can be dangerous because your lower back may go into hyperflexion as it supports your body weight in the down position, and may be hyperextended when you try to return to the upright position. In addition, your knees are frequently hyperextended in this exercise. The bouncing nature of this exercise only adds to these problems.

Standing and reaching for your toes while locking your knees may lead to both knee and back injury, and may overstretch the muscles and ligaments of the lumbar region. Charles Corbin and Ruth Lindsey warn that these exercises are especially hazardous if you suffer from back problems. In addition, Helen Timmermans and Malissa Martin report that these exercises can compress the sciatic nerve. Lorna and Peter Francis state, "Exercises involving trunk flexion in a standing position further tighten the muscles of the back and can contribute to a muscle imbalance. These exercises serve no logical purpose and in the interest of safety should be omitted from dance-exercise programs."

4. Flat back bounces

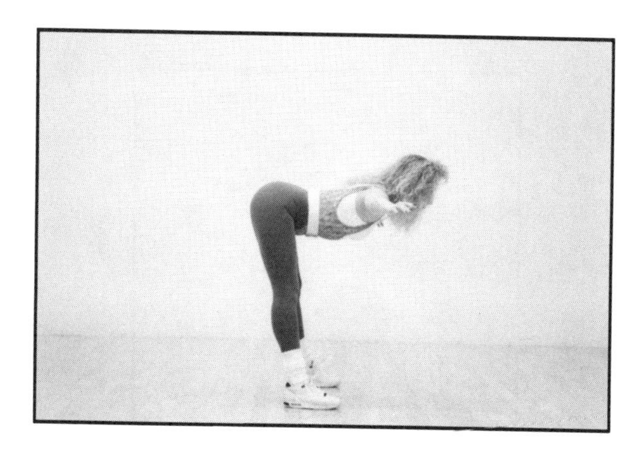

This activity is featured in many dance-exercise videos, and is performed standing with locked knees while bending at the hips with your back flat and your arms extended out to the sides. To top it off, this maneuver is frequently accompanied by a bouncing motion. This exercise is dangerous because your lower back and knees are hyperextended. Karen Clippinger-Robertson warns that compensating by slightly flexing your knees will not make this a "safe" exercise.

5. Ballet barre (hamstring) stretches

According to Charles Corbin and Ruth Lindsey, when performing ballet barre exercises, your lower back is put at risk of injury when you extend your leg 90 degrees or more above the supporting leg, while bending your

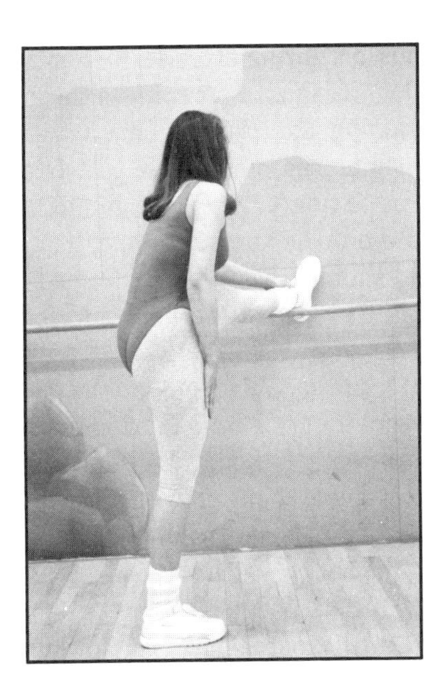

upper body over the extended leg. This may also lead to *pyriformis* syndrome (irritation of a muscle located deep in the buttocks) and sciatic-nerve pain.

SAFE EXERCISE GUIDELINES

There are several points to consider to protect your lower back from injury when you are participating in an exercise program.

According to Lorna and Peter Francis, the key to good back fitness is to make sure that "tight muscles are continually stretched and weaker muscles are carefully strengthened." Generally, this means stretching the hip flexors, hamstrings, and lower-back muscles while strengthening the abdominals.

Always keep your knees slightly flexed. Do not hyperextend (lock) the knees.

Avoid hyperextension of (overarching) your lower back. Be aware of the role strong abdominals play in helping to flatten your lower back by keeping your pelvis straight, rather than tilted forward. Always be aware of your abdominal muscles during exercise; try to maintain good posture by keeping your abdominals in. Don't confuse this motion with holding your breath when straining. Exercises that may exaggerate the curvature of your lower back should be modified to alleviate undue strain. For example, in exercises that normally require you to raise both arms overhead, you should raise only one arm at a time.

Sit-ups or curl-ups should always be performed with bent knees to keep your lower back flat against the floor and force the abdominals, rather than the hip flexors, to do the work. Carole Zebas has stated, "When the abdominals contract, they pull on the front of the pelvis, and in so doing, they prevent the back from moving inward," reducing stress to your lower back. According to Len Kravitz and Susan Kutner, "Strong abdominals can, for example, help prevent the vertebral column from being continually hyperextended as seen in the anterior pelvic tilt (pelvis tilts forward, arching the back), which is the most common misalignment seen among dance-exercise students."

Finally, maintain flexibility of the hip flexor, lower back, and hamstring muscle groups by frequently performing stretching exercises (as described in the next section).

SAFE ALTERNATIVES

The Hamstrings

1. The sit-and-reach exercise

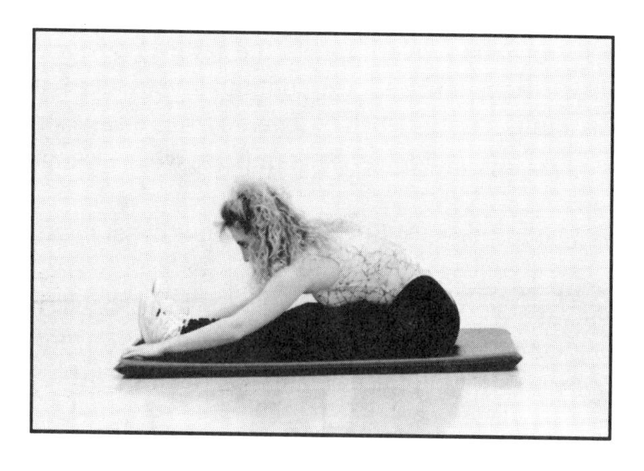

Sit with your legs extended forward and your knees flat, but not hyperextended. Gradually reach forward for your toes, bending from your hips rather than your waist.

2. The modified knee hug

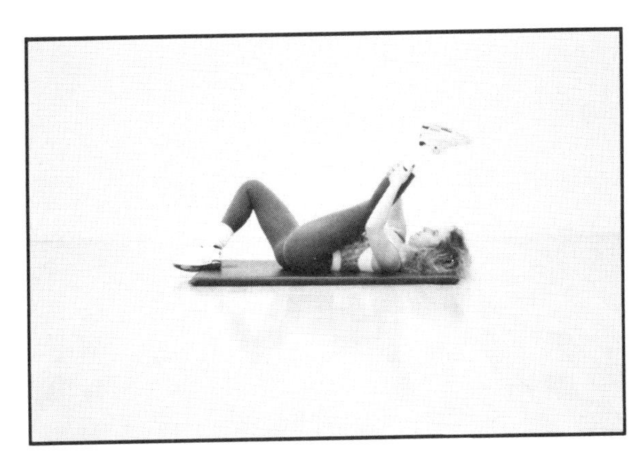

Lie on your back with your right leg bent and your right foot flat on the floor. Bring your left knee toward your chest and grasp your left leg with your hands behind the thigh. Now try to straighten the leg. Do not bring the leg to a position of hyperextension, but keep your knee flexed while gently pulling your leg toward your chest to reach a static (nonmoving) stretch. You may move your hands up toward your left calf as flexibility increases. This exercise is designed to stretch both your hamstrings and lower back.

3. The modified hurdler's stretch

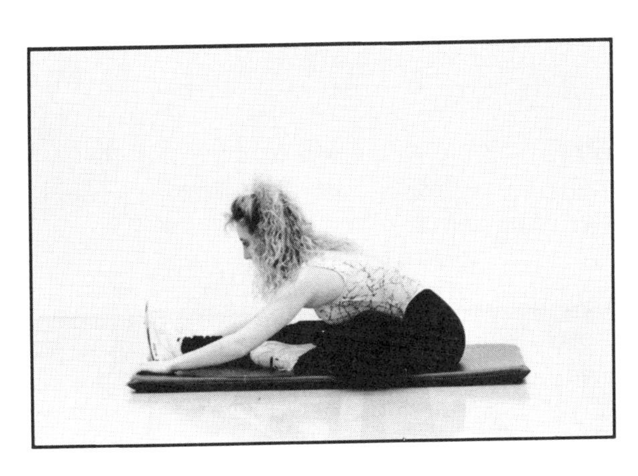

Sit with your right leg extended in front of you and your left leg bent, resting the sole of the left foot next to your right knee or inside of your right thigh. Bend forward from the hip, keeping your chest and head up while reaching forward for a static stretch. Be careful that the bent knee is not forced into hyperflexion or severely twisted.

The Lower-Back Muscles

1. *One-leg stretcher (stretches the hamstrings and the lower back)*

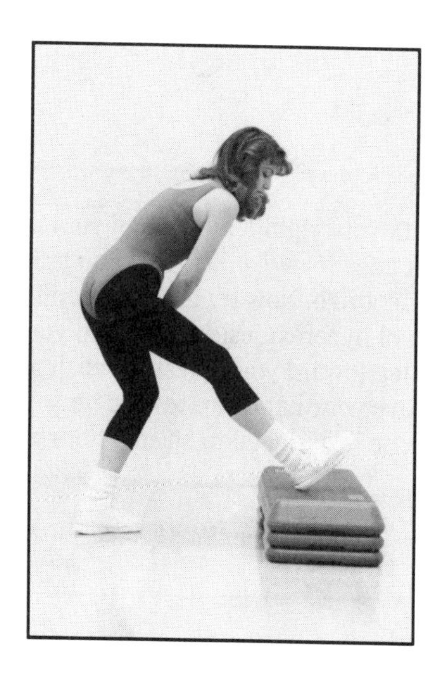

Stand with your right leg on a low bench, pushing the heel against it. Then, try to touch your head to your right knee. Be sure to keep both knees slightly flexed. Repeat with the left leg.

2. *One-leg knee hug*

Lie on your back. With both hands on the back of your left thigh just below the knee, pull your leg toward your chest. As you pull, you can lift your head off the floor to an upright position if you desire. Change legs. You can receive the additional benefit of stretching your hip flexors by stabilizing your straight leg.

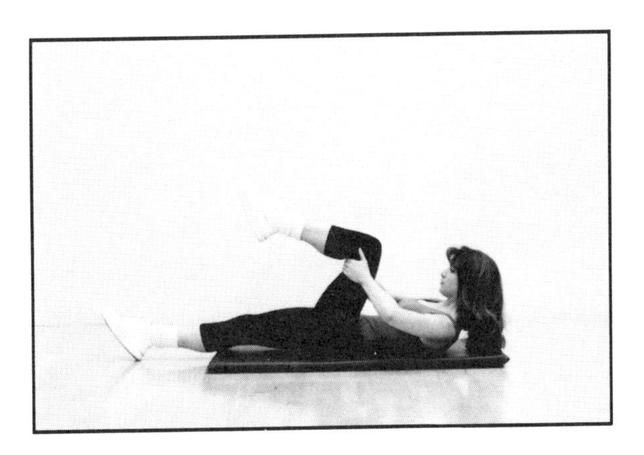

3. *The knee hug*

Peter and Lorna Francis explain that "to stretch tight back muscles, lie on your back and grasp your thighs. Pull your thighs to your chest, relax, and breathe normally while you are stretching." Be sure to grasp behind your thighs rather than over your knees when performing this exercise.

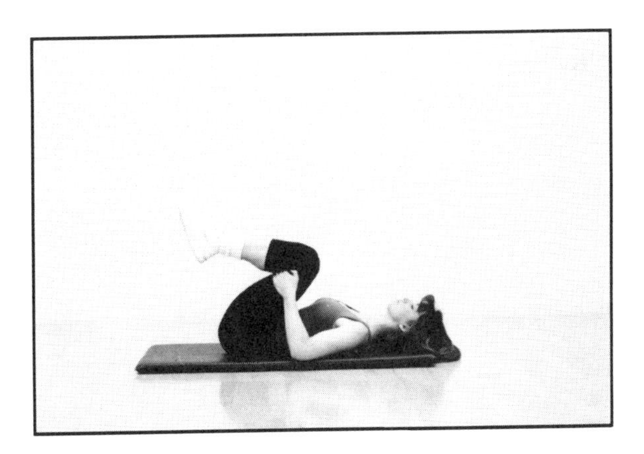

4. Cat and camel

Begin on your hands and knees with your abdomen relaxed and back curving downward, head up. Now tighten your stomach muscles and arch your back upward, allowing the head to drop and follow the arch of the back naturally.

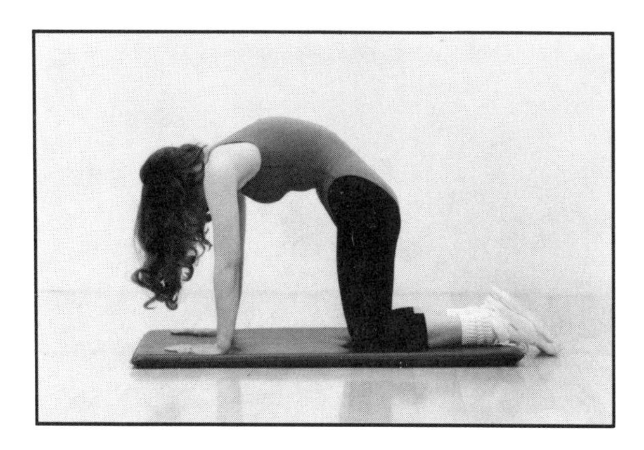

Iliopsoas *Muscles (Hip Flexors)*

1. Standing position

Place one foot ahead of the other, keeping both feet flat on the floor and parallel. Push your hips forward by curling the pelvis under. The knees may be slightly bent. You should feel tension in the quadriceps of the front leg and the inner thigh and hip flexors of the back leg.

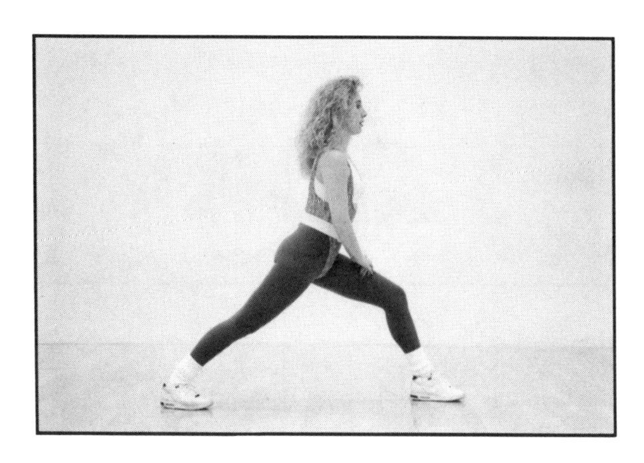

2. Kneeling position

Resting on your forearms, kneel on your left leg to form a 90-degree angle, keeping your left knee and ankle in a straight line at all times, while lifting and stretching your right leg backward. Press your hips forward and downward. Tension should be felt as in the standing position.

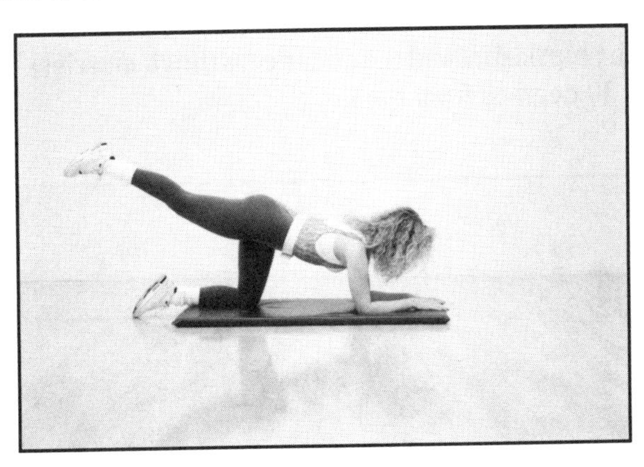

Abdominal Muscles

Karen Clippinger-Robertson explains that abdominal strength is key for preventing lower-back pain, and is important both to correct the common postural problem of *lumbar lordosis* (sway back) and to prevent lower-back injury. The following exercises will improve abdominal strength and endurance.

1. Pelvic tilt

Lying on your back with your knees bent, pull the abdominals in while pushing your lower back to the floor. Hold for six to eight counts and release. Repeat several times. Do not hold your breath.

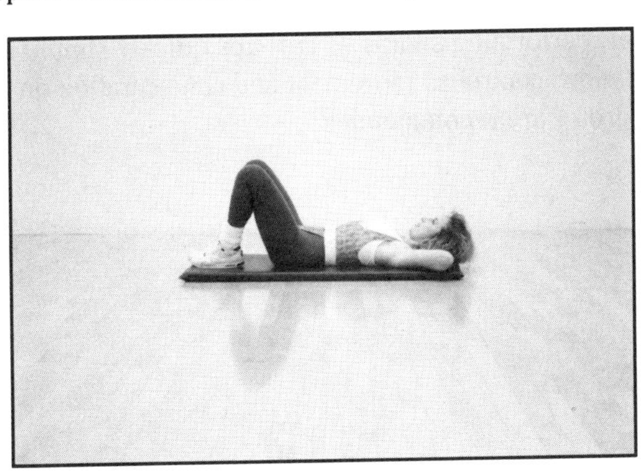

2. *Curl-ups*

Pull in your abdominal muscles to tighten and flatten the abdominal region. Press your back to the floor. Then, curl your chin to your chest and "curl-up." Reverse ("curl-down"), keeping the abdominals pulled in tight and flat. Keep your knees bent with your heels 16 to 18 inches from the hips. Do not perform curl-ups with your feet held down, which tends to activate the hip flexors and the quadriceps (thigh muscles). You should only rise to 30 degrees from the floor.

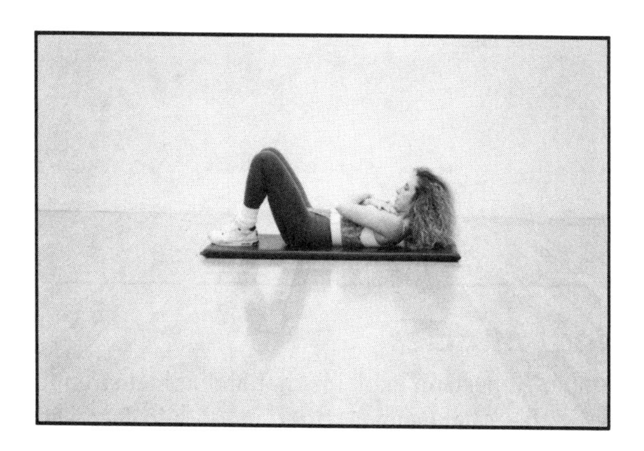

Keep your hands at the side of your head or on your shoulders, rather than locked behind your head. In this position you won't be tempted to pull on your head and neck to help yourself up, while still providing support for your head. Keeping your arms at the side of your legs or crossing them over your chest makes curling-up easier. Until you build enough strength to keep your hands at the side of your head, you may use these other positions.

Remember, performing sit-ups or curl-ups quickly should not be your goal. Rather, slow, controlled movement and concentration on the abdominal muscle group are recommended.

3. *Crunch rotations*

Begin lying on your back with your legs bent and elevated, resting on a chair or equipment of similar height. Slowly curl-up until your abdominal muscles are fully contracted.

Len Kravitz and Susan Kutner suggest adding a slight variation by lifting the right shoulder blade off the floor as you curl-up and twisting to the left side. Reverse. This variation exercises more of the abdominal muscles.

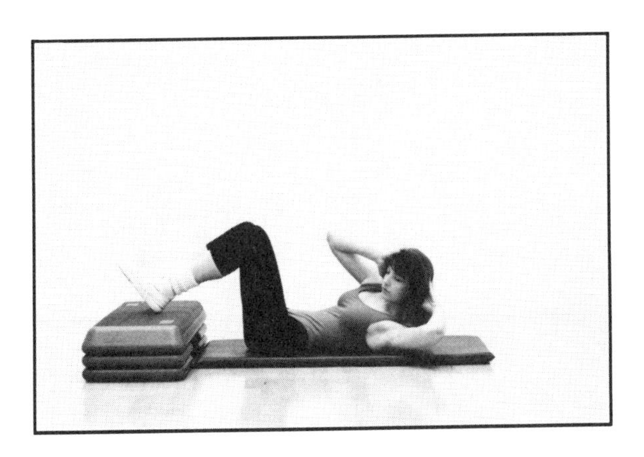

MODIFICATIONS FOR SOME QUESTIONABLE EXERCISES

1. *Hands and knees on the floor*

Place your elbows on the floor instead of your hands. Keep your abdominals pulled in tight to help flatten and stabilize your lower back. If performing leg lifts, lift your leg only to hip height so that you keep a straight line from head to toe (don't arch your back). Perform this exercise slowly and maintain control.

2. Hamstring stretch at the ballet barre

Lower the barre so your foot is not raised above a 90-degree angle, and flex your knee slightly. Holding your foot in a position above 90 degrees can lead to sciatica.

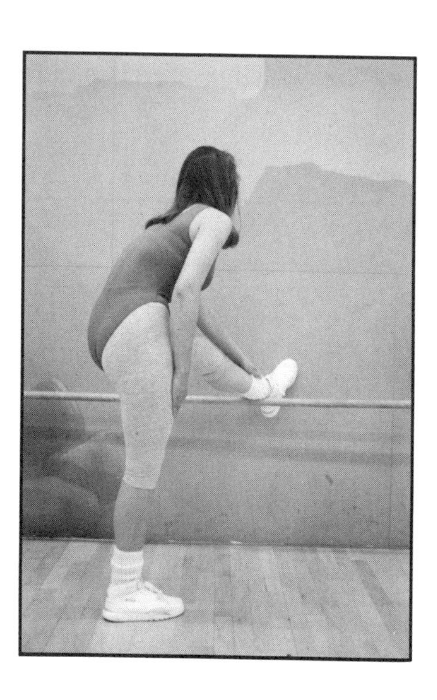

SUMMARY

A combination of strengthening exercises for the abdominals and flexibility exercises for the hip-flexor, lower-back, and hamstring muscles will guard against back pain. Avoid exercises that cause hyperextension (arching) of the lower back. Avoid placing undue strain on the back by using caution when performing forward-flexion exercises, particularly ones that incorporate a twisting motion as in windmill toe touches.

Be constantly aware of your posture in daily activities and during exercise. Concentrate on keeping your abdominals pulled in tight and your lower back flat as you exercise. Cushion your movements by flexing your ankle, knee, and hip joints.

NINE

TAKE IT ON THE HIP!

Hip Exercises

The hip is an often ignored but occasionally injured area of the body. Hip exercises are performed rarely by the general population, but play a major role in aerobics classes. In order to help guard against hip injury, it is important to exercise the muscles at all joints that enhance hip stability. Many of these are two-joint muscles, i.e., they cross both the hip and knee joints. The muscles of the hip region that are of particular concern are the *adductor magnus, adductor longus, adductor brevis, gluteus maximus, rectus femoris, iliacus,* and *psoas major*. These last two muscles flex the hip joint.

The group of muscles that make up the buttocks have three different functions: to extend and rotate the thighs and to move the legs. The *gluteus maximus* is the large muscle lying just under the skin that shapes the buttocks. It works to extend the thigh. The *gluteus medius* and *minimus* are located toward the outside of the buttocks and primarily work to move the leg sideways (abduction). The *gluteus medius* also works as an extensor and rotator of the thigh. In addition to these muscles, there is a group of six relatively small muscles that rotate the thigh to the outside. Deborah Ellison suggests that by performing exercises that utilize these movements, the buttock muscles are toned and strengthened. This will help to stabilize the hip.

Most aerobics programs include a floor-exercise routine devoted to muscle strengthening and toning exercises. Hip exercises are often included in these routines because most exercisers believe that these exercises will reduce the size of their hips. Remember, performing exercises using a specific muscle group (such as the hip muscles) will not diminish the fatty layer that has built up in that area. A combination of aerobic activity and eating a healthy diet is the best way to reduce fat. Even then, you cannot choose where the fat will be reduced. Strengthening the hip muscles will have a cosmetic benefit, because you will increase muscle tone. There is no health benefit from hip exercises such as that received by performing abdominal-strengthening exercises.

Avoid or Modify These Exercises

Avoiding exercises that put the hip into positions of undue stress will reduce the risk of hip injury. Frequently in aerobic dance-exercise classes, these positions are assumed when performing floor exercises.

1. Sidelying position with the hips flexed to 90 degrees

Holding your legs straight, raise each leg from a sidelying position. This exercise places undue stress on the rotator muscle groups of the hip (six small muscles set deep in the hip), causing muscle spasms and sciatic-nerve pain. The sidelying leg raises should be executed with your knee bent at a right angle to keep the resistance to a reasonable load. Remember, however, there is no reason to overtrain these typically overworked muscles.

2. Any hip exercise that causes you to hyperextend your back

An example would be the fire hydrant (see Chapter 8). This exercise is performed on all-fours, often leading you to arch your lower back in an attempt to compensate for poor hip strength. This may not only overstress the hip rotators, but it also puts the lower back at risk.

SAFE EXERCISE GUIDELINES

Some exercises will help create the contour and definition of the hips that you desire. It is important, however, to know which muscles to work. The muscles that flex the hip do not really need to be worked for cosmetic reasons. They are exercised adequately through daily walking, and lower-back pain can occur if they become overly developed in relation to the abdominals. You probably need to stretch the hip flexors and strengthen the abdominals rather than strengthen the hip flexors.

The other hip muscles can be exercised in a number of different ways, depending on your body position. According to Deborah Ellison:

> At the hip, the function of the muscles change dramatically depending on how much the hip is flexed. The abductors bring your leg out to the side when the leg is stationary. The external rotators normally turn the thigh outward. However, when the hip is flexed to 90 degrees (as in sitting, the hands-and-knees position, or the sidelying-L position), the rotators actually change their function and become abductors! Because of the muscles' line of pull, the *gluteus medius* and *minimus* can no longer abduct so the sideward movement is taken over by the external rotators. If you compare the size of the rotators to the *gluteus medius* and *minimus*, you will understand why exercises in these positions are more difficult—the rotators are not designed to lift such heavy loads.

She adds further that to correctly exercise the abductors, the hip must stay straight or be bent only slightly. The abductors are most efficiently worked when you are standing. The following section contains several lower-risk hip exercises.

Hands-and-Knees Position

When performing buttock exercises in this position, maintain proper alignment. The abdominals should be pulled in tight to help flatten your lower back. Do not allow your lower back to arch. Pinch your buttocks together and distribute your weight evenly on both hands (or elbows) and the opposite knee. You may support your body weight on your elbows rather than your hands to prevent arching your back. You may even try stretching your arms out flat along the floor while keeping your chest near the floor.

1. Single leg lifts from the all-fours position

When performing single leg lifts, lift your leg no higher than your hip to prevent arching of your lower back.

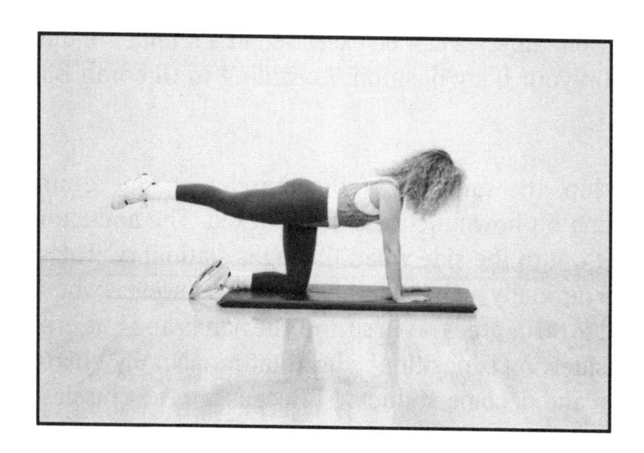

2. Single leg lifts

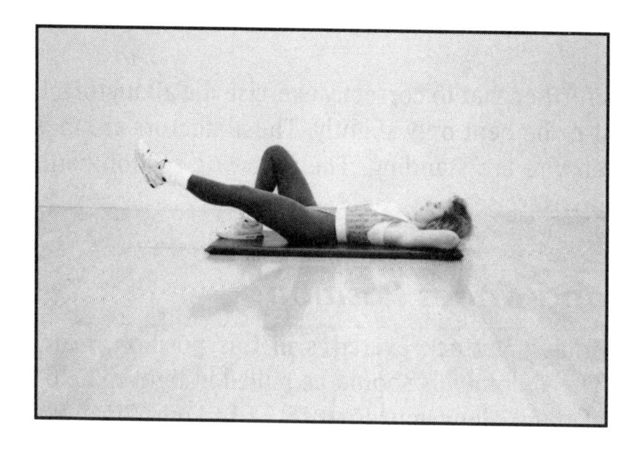

3. Modified donkey kick

Start with your thigh parallel to the floor and your knee bent at a 90-degree angle. Keep your foot flexed and lift it toward the ceiling.

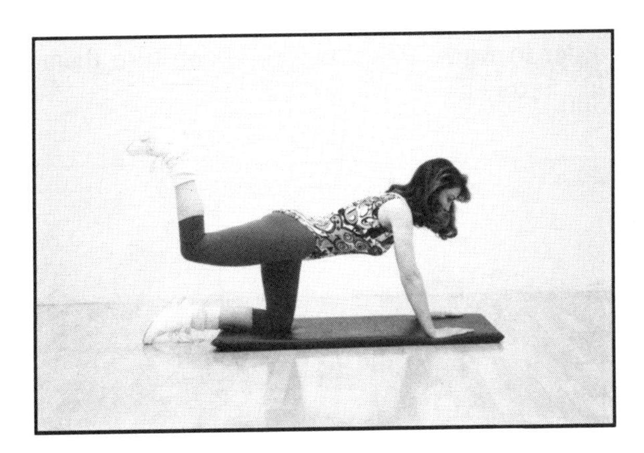

4. Knee-to-nose touch with leg extensions

From a hands-and-knees position, pull one knee toward your nose (or close to it) and then extend your leg backward horizontally. This is not a leg lift.

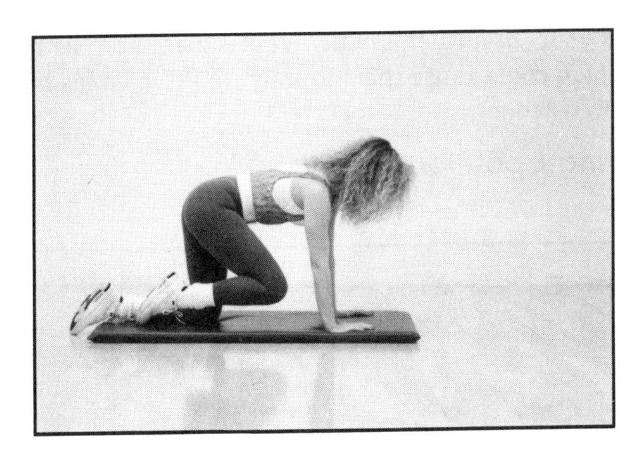

Sidelying Position

1. Side leg raises from a sidelying position

When raising your leg when you are lying on your side, take care that your pelvis does not rotate backward. Keep your knee and foot facing forward in order to work the abductors. If you turn them toward the ceiling, the hip flexors do the work.

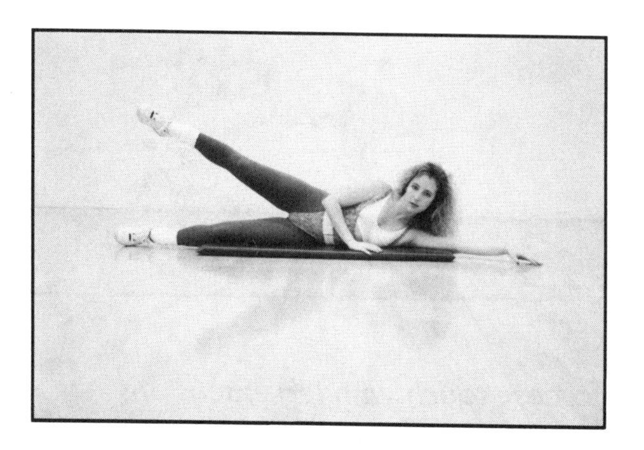

When lowering your leg, stop the downward motion when your leg forms a straight line with your hip (about 8 to 12 inches from the floor). This protects the hip joint and is particularly important for older women. If you lower your leg further, undue stress is placed on the bones of the hip joint, which could cause them to fracture if the bones have become brittle due to osteoporosis.

2. Sidelying L position

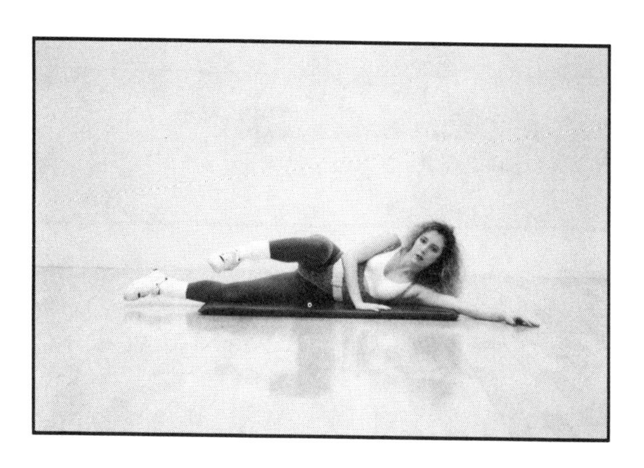

When you are exercising with your hips bent to a 90-degree angle, the rotator muscles work as abductors. Remember that these are relatively small muscles, and care must be taken not to overwork them. Bend your knee at a right angle when performing leg lifts, rather than holding your leg straight, and do not work to the point of pain. Deborah Ellison states that keeping the knee bent lowers the resistance to a reasonable load.

Standing Position

1. Standing side leg lifts

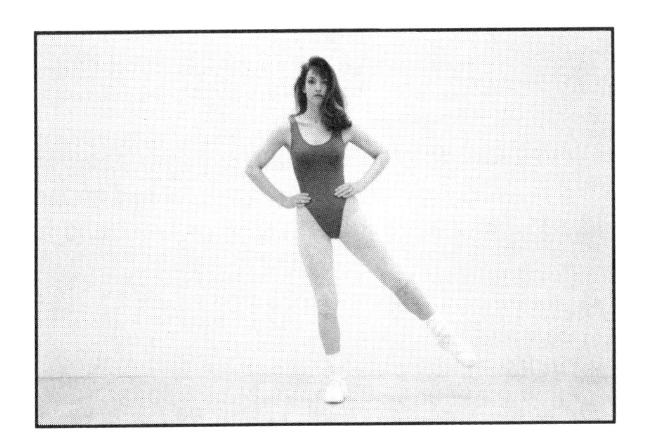

This is the most efficient exercise for working the *gluteus medius* and *minimus,* because both sides can be worked at the same time. While standing, lift one leg to the side to about 45 degrees. Be sure to keep the foot flexed with your toe pointed forward (if your toe points to the side in the direction of the lift, your hip flexors are worked). Keep the abdominals contracted and your upper body straight.

2. Forward lunges

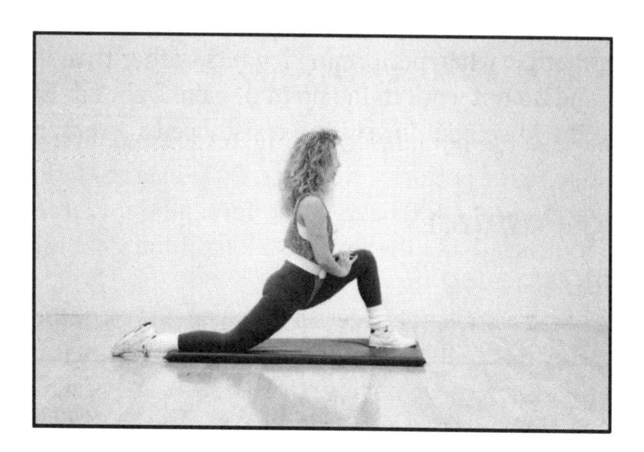

Step forward with your left foot while touching the opposite knee to the floor if possible. Be very careful to bend the left knee no more than 90 degrees, and keep it in a straight line with your ankle and foot.

On the Mat

1. Buttock tucks

Lie on your back with your knees bent. Tilt the pelvis up while squeezing the buttocks together. Be extremely careful to keep your lower back on the floor.

2. Cannonball

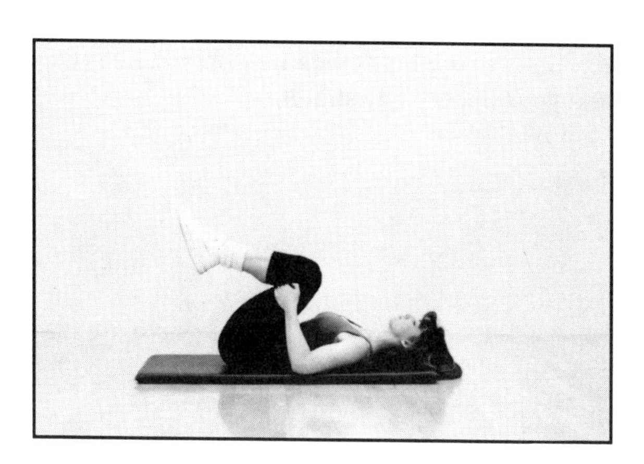

Peter and Lorna Francis suggest that: "To stretch tight back muscles, lie on your back and grasp your thighs. Pull your thighs to your chest, relax, and breathe normally while you are stretching."

SUMMARY

Exercises that use the hip muscles will help tone and strengthen them, giving definition to the buttocks. However, these exercises will not reduce the underlying layer of fat. Be sure to perform all the exercises with the abdominals contracted and the lower back flat (don't arch it) to protect your lower back.

Remember that pain is not necessary for benefits to occur. If it hurts, you need to stop, relax, stretch, and then, if the pain disappears, continue the exercise. If it remains, do not exercise. See your physician. Pain is the body's way of telling you that you are hurting it and causing injury; listen to it!

TEN

THEY SHOOT HORSES, DON'T THEY?

Knee Exercises

Knee injury is a common problem for aerobic dancers. As with most other dance-exercise injuries, James Garrick contends that much knee injury may be linked to overuse or inappropriate use. The knee injury most frequently reported is *chondromalacia patella,* a degenerative process that results in a softening of the back of the knee cap that can result in anterior knee pain.

The general consensus in the sportsmedicine community is that the best way to protect the knee is by strengthening the surrounding musculature. The major areas of concern in the anatomy of the knee are the muscles of the *quadriceps* group (front of the thigh), the hamstring group (back of the thigh), and the *gastrocnemius* (calf muscle). In addition, protection of the medial *meniscii,* the collateral (external) and cruciate (internal) ligaments, and the cartilage are important.

As with many of the other parts of the body discussed in this book, the knee is frequently injured by forcing it into positions of hyperflexion and hyperextension. These positions increase the likelihood of overstretching the ligaments that are designed to hold together the bones that constitute the knee joint.

Avoid or Modify These Exercises

To reduce the risk of knee injury, positions of extreme hyperextension and hyperflexion at the knee joint should be avoided. Additionally, avoid exercises that overstress the knee, such as those where an external load is applied.

Hyperextension of the Knee

1. Standing toe touches

When you are standing and reaching for your toes, there is a tendency to hyperextend your knees. Charles Corbin and Ruth Lindsey report that this movement may overstretch the muscles, ligaments, joint capsule, and cartilage of the knee.

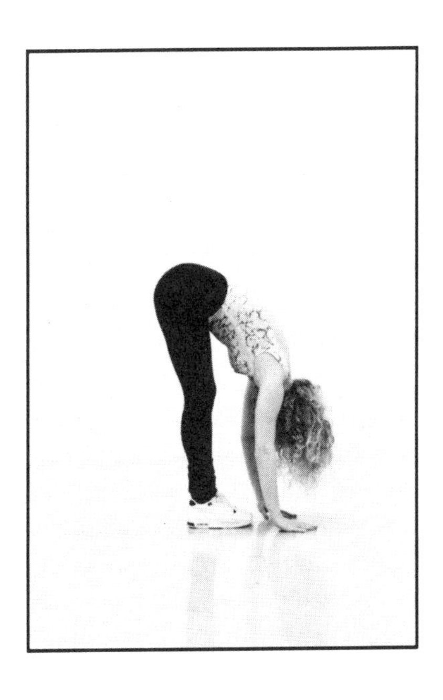

2. *Ballet barre stretch*

When you perform the ballet barre stretch, both of your knees may be placed into a position of hyperextension, which can be further aggravated by bouncing when you are in this position. Bouncing in the stretch may damage the ligaments of the knee and the cartilage.

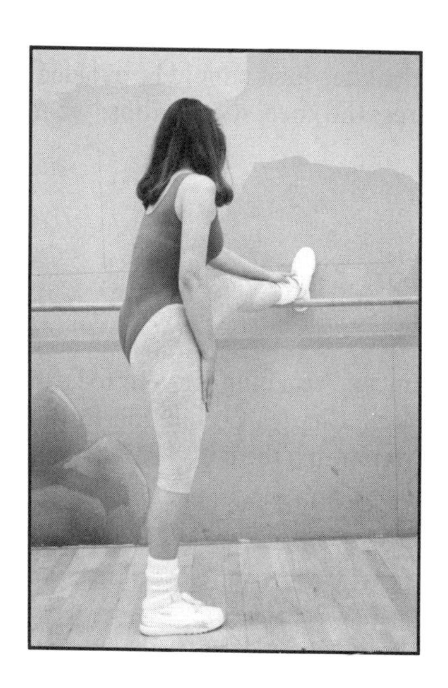

Hyperflexion of the Knee

1. *Full squats or deep knee bends*

According to Charles Corbin and Ruth Lindsey, this exercise may harm the knee joint by stretching the ligaments and irritating the synovial membrane (the membrane lining the capsule of the knee joint). Daniel Arnheim adds that forcefully bending the knees in a full-squat position may overly stretch internal (cruciate) ligaments of the knee joint.

Deep knee bends are usually performed to stretch and strengthen the quadriceps. They are similar to full squats, although full squats are usually performed while holding weights. The ligaments of the knee are at most risk when you are at the lowest point of a deep knee bend, when a shift of force from the quadriceps to the patellar ligaments occurs. Carol Teitz has reported that patellofemoral force is as high as 7.6 times body weight at this point during a deep knee bend, which is excessive force for a joint to handle when it is in a position of weakness.

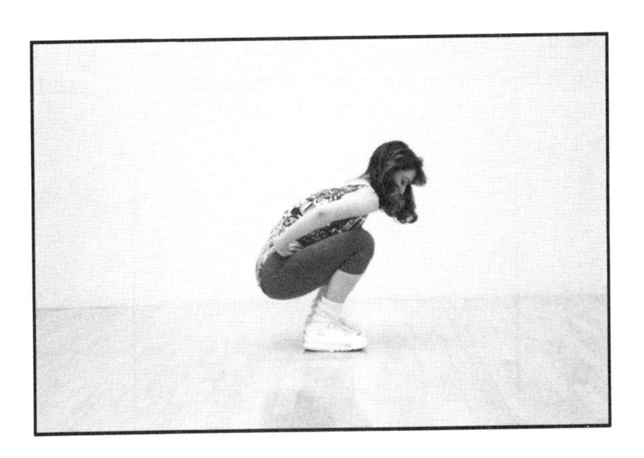

2. *Squat thrusts*

Squat thrusts, similar to full squats and deep knee bends, place additional stress on the knee because they begin with a jump into position. Charles Corbin and Ruth Lindsey warn that both the ligaments and the cartilage of the knee are placed at risk when you perform this exercise.

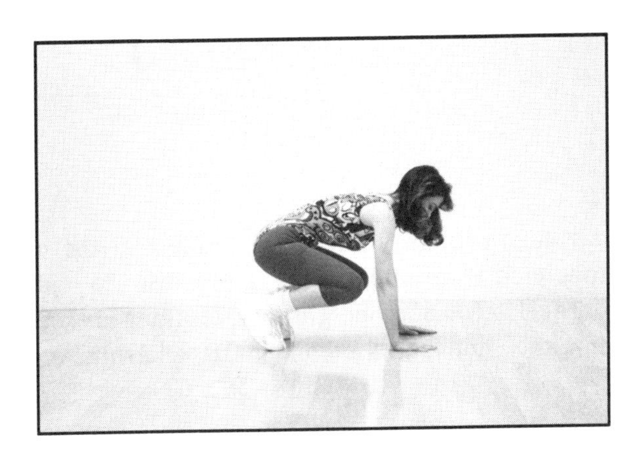

3. Pliés

The *plié* has its origins in ballet. In ballet, a *plié* consists of flexion at the hips, knees, and ankles, while keeping the torso straight. According to Daniel Arnheim, if the *plié* is performed incorrectly, it can produce severe stress on the inner aspects of the knee. This may potentially accentuate or even cause knock-knees, promote pronation (rolling inward) of your foot, and lower the arch of your foot. Carol Teitz claims that even minor aberrations in *plié* technique, repeated over time, may produce clinical problems.

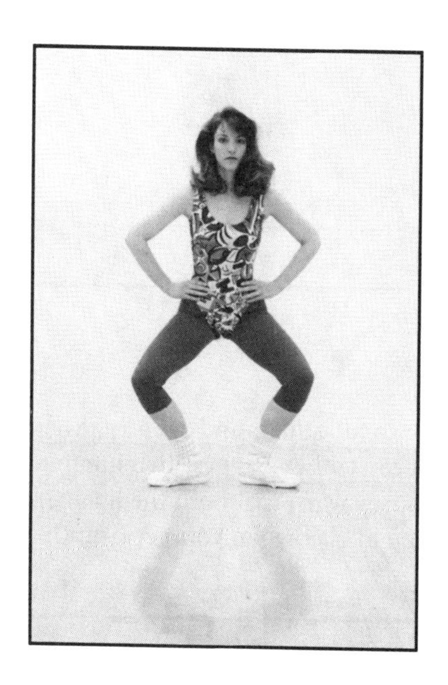

4. Turnout

Turnout is a rotation of the entire leg beginning at the hips. Karen Clippinger-Robertson reports that many of the overuse injuries occurring in dance are related to improper turnout, resulting in excessive stress at the back, hip, knee, and foot. According to Daniel Arnheim, if you force your feet to turn out while rotating the knees inward you may create rotational stress at the knee, misalign the kneecaps, and cause a roughness on the surface of the patella (knee cap).

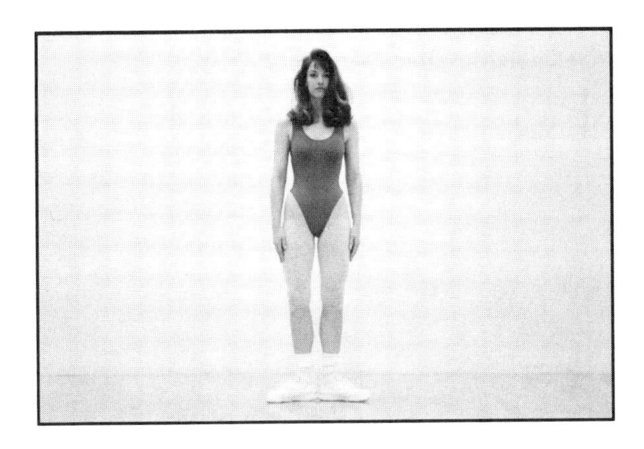

5. Hurdler's stretch

The hurdler's stretch is performed by sitting on the ground with one leg straight in front of your body and the other bent to the side in a hurdling position. Charles Corbin and Ruth Lindsey report that this position is risky because it may strain the groin, weaken the medial ligament of the bent knee, and put great stress on the cartilage of the bent knee.

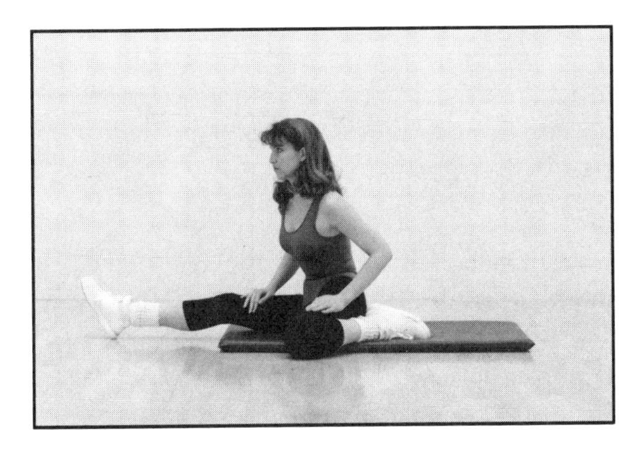

6. Shin stretches

This exercise consists of folding your feet under and sitting back so that your buttocks rest on your heels. Shin and quadriceps stretches can be dangerous when the knee is hyperflexed 120 degrees or more. Charles Corbin and Ruth Lindsey suggest that this may damage the knee by tearing the cartilage or by stretching the ligaments.

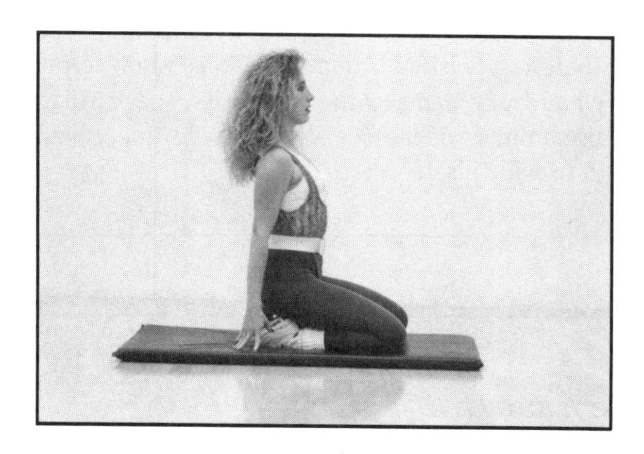

7. Knee to chest, hands over knee

Lie on your back, bending your left leg at the knee and placing your hands over and slightly below your knee. Then pull your knee toward your chest.

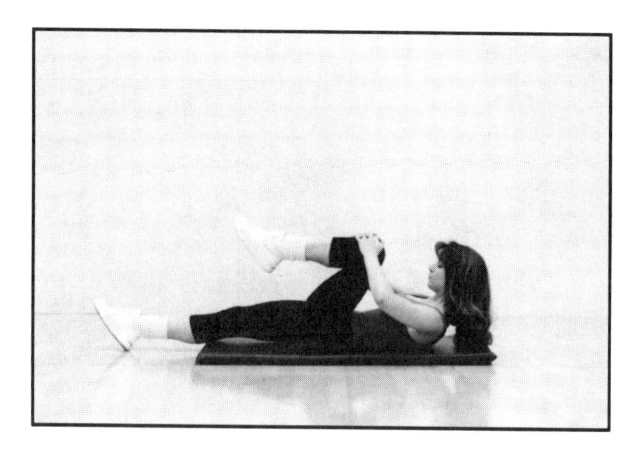

The knee-to-chest exercise can be beneficial in improving hamstring flexibility. However, when you attempt to pull your knee in closer to your chest, you may actually pull it into a state of hyperflexion. This most commonly occurs when you place your hands over the knee and pull on it.

8. Heel to buttock

The heel-to-buttock exercise is performed by standing on one foot and pulling the toe of the opposite foot toward your buttock. It is designed to stretch the quadriceps. Karen Smith explains that when you reach back and pull your toe in toward your buttock, hyperflexion occurs. To confound this situation, a twisting action at the knee often accompanies this movement, which may damage the ligaments, the cartilage, and the *meniscii*. Maintaining a wider angle at the knee by not pulling as hard on the toe would provide a safer alternative.

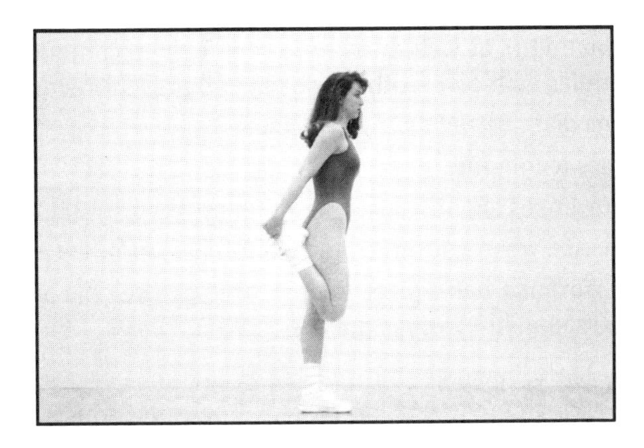

9. Duck walk

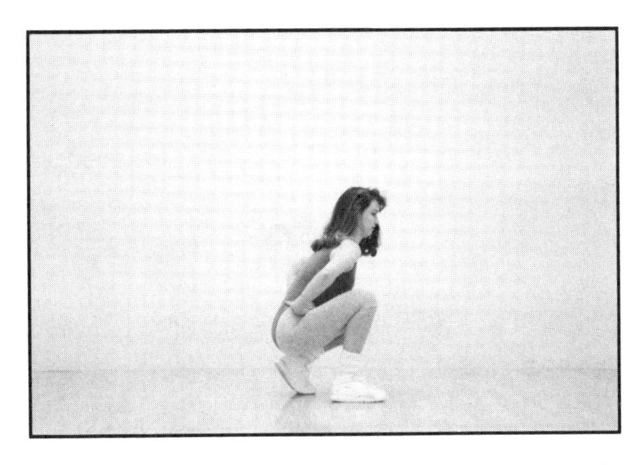

The duck walk was once used as a conditioning exercise by the military; it is now used for punishment and as a form of torture! This movement involves squatting with your hands on your hips, your buttocks low, and your knees pointing up. While in this squatting position, you attempt to walk without straightening your knees, causing extreme flexion. This is one exercise that should be avoided completely.

SAFE EXERCISE GUIDELINES

To help guard against injury to the knee, Daniel Arnheim and others suggest the following guidelines:

1. Use preventive conditioning. Make sure that the muscles that stabilize the joint are strong. According to Carol Teitz, for most knee problems, *vastus-medialis* strengthening (the muscle located at the inner, lower part of the thigh), as well as correction of faulty technique and training schedules, will correct the problem and prevent recurrence.
2. Seek immediate care if an injury occurs.
3. Use proper technique.
4. Keep your knees slightly flexed at all times when stretching.
5. Don't bounce when your knees are in full flexion or extension.
6. When performing half-squats, keep your knee over the ankle, pointing in the same direction as the toes.

Safe Alternatives

1. Hands under knee for knee hug

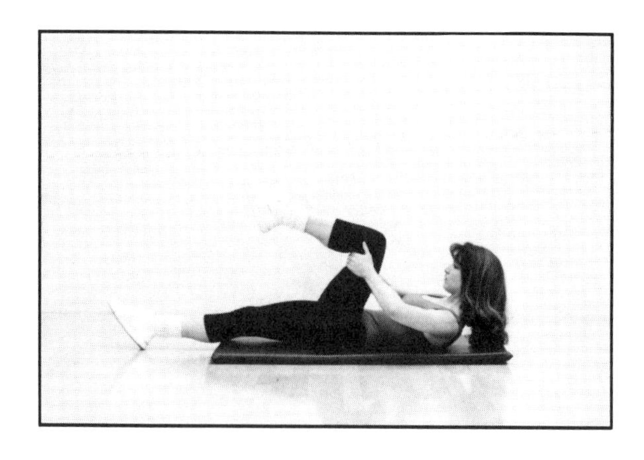

Charles Corbin and Ruth Lindsey have suggested this position as a safe alternative to the standard knee hug. In this exercise your hands are placed behind your leg instead of over the knee, reducing the stress placed on the knee joint.

2. *Sit and reach*

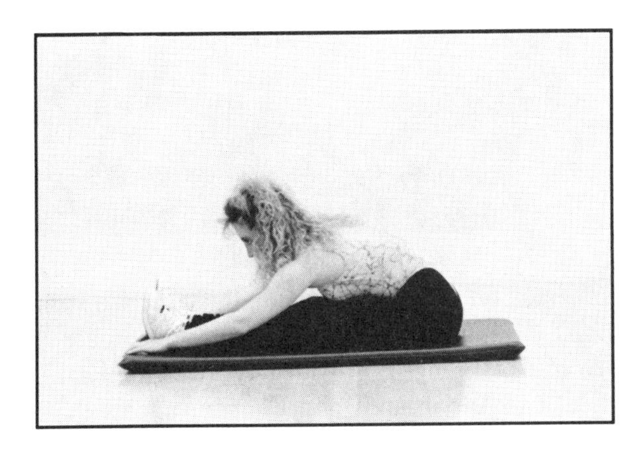

Sit with your legs straight out in front of your body, and slowly lean forward from your hips while reaching for your toes. Keep your knees slightly flexed.

3. *V-sit*

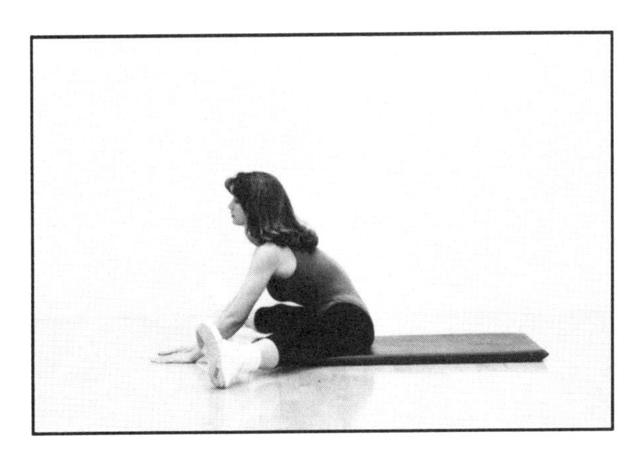

Sit with your legs parted in a V-shape, slightly bending your knees. Now, slowly lean forward from the hips.

4. Leg extensions

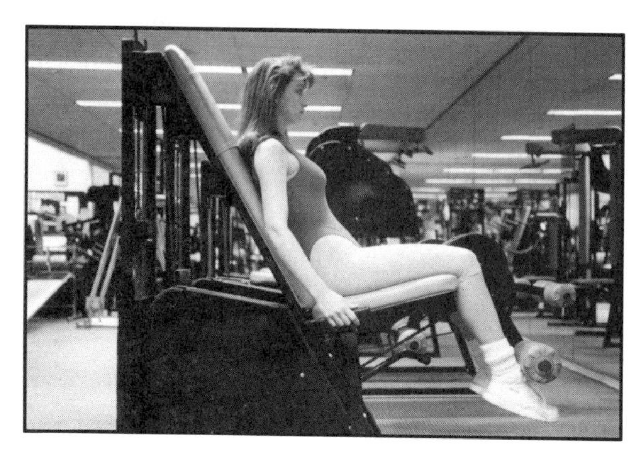

Typically performed on a weight machine, this exercise strengthens the *vastus medialis.* Sitting on the machine with your knees bent, extend your legs forward. Resistance is provided by a weighted bar that rests on your shins. Marlene Adrian and John Cooper suggest that many knee injuries can be avoided by flexing the foot and fully extending the knee when performing the leg extension.

SUMMARY

The knee is a multifunctional joint, allowing us to perform a variety of activities. Protection of our knees is critical to maintain our freedom of movement. There are many safe exercises that strengthen and improve the flexibility of the musculature of the legs without damaging the knee. Carol Teitz reminds us that, "Relative malalignment of the lower extremities will predispose the dancer to patellofemoral problems, but in the vast majority of cases, either faulty technique or overuse are to blame."

ELEVEN

FEET DON'T FAIL ME NOW

Lower Leg, Ankle, and Foot Exercises

Most dance-exercise injuries occur to the foot, ankle, shin, lower back, and knee, most of which can be attributed to overuse. However, poor technique may compound the effects of overtraining. There are many additional causes of foot injuries including: exercising on hard surfaces, improper foot protection, changing surfaces, anatomical imbalance, and excessive supination (rolling out) or pronation (rolling in). If we consider the fact that the lower leg acts as a link system, meaning that a stress applied to one part usually affects the other parts, we can see how improper positioning of your foot may lead to problems in the entire lower body.

WHAT ARE THE MOST COMMON LOWER-LEG AND FOOT PROBLEMS?

Shinsplints

Shinsplints is a term used to describe any general pain or discomfort in the shin. Both Douglas Ritchie and Lorna Francis and their colleagues report that shin pain is the most commonly reported aerobic-dance injury. There are at least six different clinical injuries that people commonly call "shinsplints." Because of this, general recommendations are difficult to give for treating this problem. Each injury should be treated individually. The factors contributing to shinsplint formation include muscular imbalance, overuse, poor technique, improper footwear, poor surface, and lack of or poorly performed warmups.

Plantar Fasciitis

The *plantar fascia* is a thick piece of tissue that is attached to the heel bone as a narrow band, which then broadens as it runs toward the base of the toes. According to Len Kravitz, collapse of the arch structure places considerable strain on this tissue and is a common cause of arch and heel pain. Studies by Douglas Ritchie and Lorna Francis and their colleagues show that *plantar fasciitis* is the second most common dance-exercise injury.

Stress Fracture

A stress fracture is a hairline crack in the bone typically brought on by overtraining. If left untreated, this crack may develop into a larger fracture.

Sprains

Sprains involve an overstretching of the ligaments supporting the ankle, usually caused by either pronating or supinating. A sprain is a traumatic injury, or one that occurs suddenly, such as when you twist your ankle.

AVOID OR MODIFY THESE EXERCISES

Unlike injuries to other parts of the body, most lower-leg, ankle, and foot injuries are not normally caused by poor positioning. However, injury to the ankle may occur due to excessive rotation either when the ankle rolls out (supination) or when it rolls in (pronation).

Douglas Ritchie points out that factors such as type of shoe, floor surface, technique, and amount of participation may be more important in determining overall injury frequency. Perhaps the two most important causes of injury to this region are overuse and poor foot protection.

Repeatedly rising on your toes or heels may weaken the long arch of your foot. While tiptoeing exercises will develop your calf muscles, they will also stretch the muscles and ligaments that help support the long arch of your foot; walking on your heels can have the same effect. Charles Corbin and Ruth Lindsey suggest that these movements can be made safer if they are performed with the toes turned slightly in.

High-impact exercises in which you perform high, jumping motions can be dangerous. Karen Clippinger-Robertson reports that these exercises are even more risky when you land on only one foot.

If your shoes or the dance surface are too hard so that they do not absorb impact forces, your body will have to absorb these forces. Surfaces such as concrete or carpet over concrete should be avoided; poor shoes, or dancing barefoot, may also lead to leg, ankle, and foot problems. Lorna and Peter Francis and Kim Welshons-Smith warn that "the repeated impact of the dancer's feet on firm surfaces can produce overuse injuries."

SAFE EXERCISE GUIDELINES

Select proper footwear. Lorna and Peter Francis and Kim Welshons-Smith recommend that you wear shoes that provide impact protection under the metatarsal heads (balls of the feet) and that control undesirable pronation. Because of their design, running or tennis shoes are generally not suitable for aerobic dance. Similarly, you should avoid hard dance surfaces that do not absorb impact (for more on dance shoes and surfaces, see Chapter 2).

Practice proper technique. Work on balance and proper foot placement.

Avoid overtraining or overuse. Give your lower limbs adequate recovery time after a workout.

Work on symmetrical development. Don't spend the entire class working on the front portion of your foot. Allow your heel to touch the ground when performing the aerobic portion of the exercise routine. Develop both the anterior (front) and posterior (back) muscle groups of your lower legs. Most aerobics participants need to place a greater emphasis on strengthening the *anterior tibialis* muscle and stretching the calf.

Safe Alternatives

1. Towel exercises

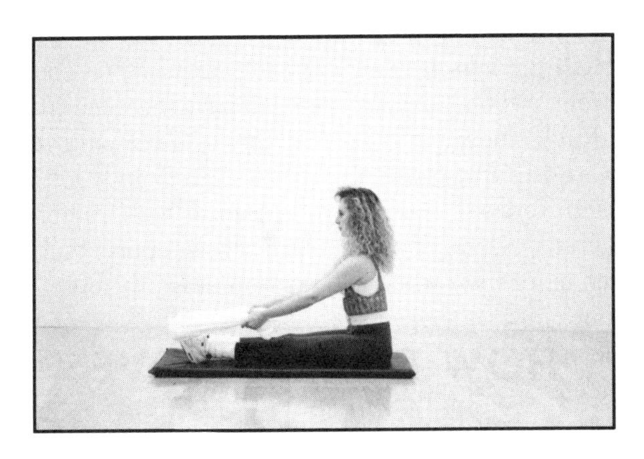

Place the towel around the ball of your foot, holding the two ends with your hands. Try to point your toes away from you as you pull on the towel to provide resistance; this will develop the calf muscles. To develop the front portion of your leg, have a partner place a towel over your toes and gently pull on it away from your body to provide resistance while you attempt to move your toes toward your knee.

2. Alphabet exercise

With your toes, try to write each letter of the alphabet in the air. Almost every possible ankle motion will be used in this exercise. To add more resistance, repeat this activity with your foot submerged in a pool or tub of water.

SUMMARY

Many lower-leg, foot, and ankle injuries can be avoided by using a little common sense. Select a safe exercise environment, proper footwear, and a rational training schedule. If pain occurs, do not try to work through it; see your physician and locate the problem.

TWELVE

HOW DO I IMPROVE MY HEART WITHOUT BREAKING IT?

Cardiovascular Exercises

The cardiovascular system must be exercised regularly to function at peak efficiency. Frequently, however, people engage in activities that put it at unnecessary risk. Effective aerobic exercise can be performed to strengthen the cardiovascular system. With cardiovascular disease being the number-one killer in the United States, it is important that the cardiovascular system receive exercise that is of sufficient frequency, intensity, and duration for optimal benefit.

Aerobic exercise can be any type of exercise that meets the guidelines to be classified as aerobic, not just aerobic dance. Many exercises are performed with the misguided assumption that they are aerobic, when in fact they are designed to build muscular endurance or strength (such as floor exercises and weight training). Any activity that can be continued for twenty minutes, that uses the large muscle masses (primarily the legs, but preferably the arms and legs), can be called aerobic.

Avoid or Modify These Exercises

1. Isometric exercises

Isometric exercises are activities in which the muscle generates tension but no movement occurs. For example, when you push against a wall you exert force, but there is no movement. It is especially important that people with hypertension (high blood pressure) and other cardiovascular diseases avoid isometric exercises. These exercises can raise blood pressure significantly and may trigger cardiovascular injury. Charles Corbin and Ruth Lindsey report that "isometric exercise has its advantages, but studies have shown it may be more dangerous to heart patients than isotonic exercise, since it may cause irregular heartbeats and a marked rise in blood pressure. Isometric exercise for preadolescents is also questionable because the growth centers in their bones may not have closed."

2. Valsalva maneuver

Exercises in which you hold your breath while straining (valsalva maneuver) can significantly raise your blood pressure. For example, many people hold their breath when lifting a heavy weight, such as a barbell. If there is a weakness in your vascular network, this can result in hemorrhaging and cardiovascular injury. It is important to remember to exhale when exerting maximal force.

3. Raising your arms above your head for an extended period of time

Raising your arms above your heart causes a significant increase in blood pressure. Your arms should not be elevated and held for more than a few (one to five) seconds. Alternately raising and lowering your arms while exercising will alleviate this problem.

4. Overtraining

Overtraining can be as dangerous as no exercise at all. Your body needs time to recover in order to adapt to the stress associated with exercise. In addition, the exercise should not overtax the cardiovascular system before it is ready to handle the exertion. Richard Norris points out another type of overtraining that can be dangerous involves trying too much too soon, or trying to continue to exercise at a high intensity when you are fatigued. Daniel Arnheim states, "The most likely times for injuries to occur are in the early stages of a new dance experience when the body is not adequately trained and in the very late periods of a dance session when chronic physical and mental tiredness make the dancer extremely vulnerable to injury."

GUIDELINES FOR SAFE AND EFFECTIVE EXERCISE

The American College of Sports Medicine (ACSM) has established guidelines for the healthy adult to achieve cardiovascular fitness, based upon the proper combination of frequency, intensity, duration, and mode of exercise.

Frequency

Aerobic exercise should be performed a minimum of three days per week to a maximum of five days per week. Exercising less than three days per week will not bring about a training effect, while exercising more than five days per week will result in small improvements in cardiovascular fitness and a greatly increased risk of injury.

Intensity

Exercise at a heart rate of 50 to 85 percent of your maximal heart-rate reserve. This can be calculated by taking your age and subtracting it from 220. Then subtract your resting heart rate and multiply it by .50 for the lower limit and .85 for the upper limit. The resting heart rate must then be added to determine the training zone.

Example: A 30-year-old exerciser with a resting heart rate of 65.

220 − 30 = 190 This is your estimated maximum heart rate.

190 − 65 = 125 This is your heart-rate reserve.

125 times .50 = 63 and 125 times .85 = 106

63 + 65 = 128 and 106 + 65 = 171

Lower limit = 128 and upper limit = 171.

Duration

The exercise session should include a minimum of twenty minutes and a maximum of sixty minutes of aerobic activity. It takes approximately twenty minutes for your body to begin to utilize fat as the primary fuel source, and this is also the threshold for significant cardiovascular benefit. Exercising more than an hour increases your risk for injury while offering only modest improvements in fitness.

Mode

Rhythmical activities utilizing your body's large muscle masses should be the focus of aerobic exercise, such as moving your legs (and possibly your arms) in a repetitive fashion for a minimum of twenty minutes. The dance portion of an aerobics class is an example of an acceptable activity.

As a side note, the ACSM recently suggested guidelines for muscular strength and endurance training. They suggest that you participate in weight training at least twice a week and perform eight to ten exercises involving the major muscle groups. One set of eight to twelve repetitions of each exercise are recommended, or until your muscles are near fatigue.

SAFETY GUIDELINES

Keep the activity rhythmical in nature. The pumping action of the muscle promotes the return of blood to the heart and keeps your blood pressure in a safe region.

Remember to exhale while exerting maximal force and refrain from holding your breath when exercising. There is no ideal breathing pattern that should be practiced; you should breathe in a rhythm that feels natural to you. The key is to continue breathing at all times.

Monitor your cardiovascular response. This can be done by monitoring heart rate or by monitoring your rating of perceived exertion. Perceived exertion is based upon your perception of how hard you are working. You should work at a level that would fall between somewhat hard and hard.

Progress gradually. Allow your body to adapt to the stresses of exercise before increasing their intensity. In fact, it is generally recommended that you increase the duration of an exercise session before adjusting intensity.

When fatigued, rest. Your body needs recovery time to function effectively. You should feel completely recovered within one hour of the termination of your exercise session.

Summary

The cardiovascular system needs regular aerobic exercise. That exercise should be performed three to five days per week and should last a minimum of twenty minutes. Listen to your body. It will tell you if you need to adjust the intensity of your exercise session. Overtraining can be as dangerous as not doing enough exercise.

III

FINISHING TOUCHES

THIRTEEN

NOW THAT IT'S OVER, IT WASN'T THAT BAD

Cooling-down

Whew! You made it! Now that the most intensive part of your workout has ended, don't ignore the important cool-down period. The purpose of cooling-down is to allow the body to return gradually to its resting state. This is best accomplished by lowering the intensity of your previous exercise program and following it up with flexibility exercises. The key to an effective cool-down is to let your body gradually adjust from its high energy output state to one of recovery.

WHEN SHOULD I COOL-DOWN?

If a floor-exercise portion is offered after your aerobic exercise, a cool-down period should be included between the aerobic segment of the workout and the floor work. In addition, a second cool-down should follow the floor-exercise portion. Generally speaking, any time that the body moves from a period of higher-intensity exercise to lower-intensity exercise, a gradual transition is recommended. This transition is what is referred to as a cool-down. The cool-down is important because it allows your body to gradually adjust to the change in exercise intensity. It will help prevent feelings of light-headedness and will shorten your recovery time.

WHAT MAKES UP THE COOL-DOWN?

The cool-down should be composed of lower-intensity general body movements followed by stretching exercises for flexibility enhancement. Karen Smith recommends that, during the cool-down, you should relax, breathe normally, avoid bouncing, and never exercise in pain.

It is during the cool-down portion of the exercise program that maximal gains in flexibility are possible. After vigorous aerobic exercise, the muscles become more pliable because they are warm, enhancing their range of motion. By performing stretching exercises now, your overall flexibility will be greatly improved. The flexibility exercises should be primarily static (nonbouncing) in nature. Each muscle should be brought into a position in which a mild stretch is felt and that position should be held for a minimum of fifteen seconds. The longer you hold a position of stretch, the greater the improvement in flexibility will be. However, because we are realistically limited by time, there must be some limit to the total time spent on stretching. Generally speaking, the cool-down portion of your aerobics class should last a minimum of ten minutes.

In addition to stretching exercises, the cool-down should involve lower-intensity general body movements designed to assist in blood flow, aid in temperature regulation, and gradually bring the body back to a resting state. Many of the same exercises that were used in the warmup can be used in reverse order in the cool-down. The cool-down should not be used to tone the muscles by working against resistance. Arm movements should be kept below shoulder level and gradually reduced in intensity. Your upper body should be kept erect during the first few minutes of the recovery. You should not perform exercises that require you to lower your head to the floor; this could cause extreme dizziness and loss of balance. Keep in mind that it is important to keep moving during the first part of the cool-down so that muscular contractions will aid the return of blood to the heart.

WHAT OCCURS DURING THE COOL-DOWN?

Because the cool-down period is primarily designed to return the body to its resting state, relaxing the muscles should be a primary focus. Exercise-physiology research teaches us that during the cool-down phase of an exercise program, some of the accumulated lactic acid (a by-product of high-intensity exercise related to fatigue) begins to be reconverted into pyruvic acid, which may eventually provide energy for further movement. The cool-down also aids in venous return, which means it helps the blood get back to the heart. Breathing rates return to normal, hormone levels are stabilized, and energy stores are replenished. The body is also cooled so that its temperature level returns to the resting state. The cool-down period has also been linked to reducing postexercise pain and stiffness.

WHAT EXERCISES SHOULD I INCLUDE IN THE COOL-DOWN?

The cool-down should include slow walking and stretching exercises that focus on the muscles that were primarily involved in your aerobic and muscular-endurance workout. You should at least stretch out the major muscle groups of the body. Most aerobic classes include a cool-down section that will stretch these muscles. Remember, it is very important that you do not skip the cool-down. Any of the exercises listed as safe alternatives in the preceding chapters may be used as part of your cool-down. A few of these exercises are:

Neck: Ear to shoulder, neck rotation, lateral neck flexion and extension
Shoulder: Pectoral stretch, wand exercise, back scratch
Back: Modified knee hug, low back stretcher, cat and camel
Hip: Single leg lifts, standing leg lifts, forward lunges
Knee: Sit and reach, V-sit, modified knee hug
Lower leg, ankle, and foot: Towel exercise, alphabet exercise

FOURTEEN

NOW THAT I KNOW IT ALL, WHAT SHOULD I DO?

Our purpose in writing this book is not to scare you away from exercising. In fact, we hope you will participate in as many different activities as your time, budget, and lifestyle allow. Aerobic dance is no more dangerous than any other form of exercise, as long as you keep in mind certain safety tips and guidelines like those outlined in this book.

Dance exercise has been criticized because of the extent of injury associated with it. However, much of the information regarding dance-exercise injury is based upon speculation. James Garrick reports that little scientific information dealing with the medical problems of aerobic dance has been available. Most of the criticism of aerobics has been based not on the fact that aerobic dance has been shown to be dangerous, but rather that it was developed and taught by those unschooled in exercise physiology, kinesiology, and medicine. As an exercise consumer, it is up to you to act as your own final safeguard against exercise-induced injury.

Avoiding injury can be boiled down to a few simple principles. Before embarking on any exercise program, you should be prescreened for any existing medical conditions that might limit your ability to exercise. Exercise in moderation; studies show that exercising more than three to five times a week for more than an hour a time does not significantly improve your overall fitness and can lead to fatigue and injury.

Before exercising, warmup properly. Low-intensity activity that involves movement patterns specific to the activity you will be performing should be undertaken for ten to fifteen minutes. Be sure your warmup is balanced with slow, nonballistic stretching. Gradually increase activity to the aerobic level and take additional time for comprehensive strength training.

Be sure to use proper technique. If you're not sure if you're doing a movement correctly, ask. If something hurts, stop and make sure you're not moving incorrectly. A qualified, professional exercise leader is important not only for showing you exactly how to execute each movement, but to monitor your overall progress, help you get the most out of your workout, and avoid injury.

Be an educated dance consumer. Continue to learn about your body and exercise. Often, we don't do a very good job of explaining our injuries to our doctors, and doctors, in turn, tend to disregard our minor complaints. Richard Norris explains that "if dancers can speak knowledgeably about the body and injuries, physicians will regard them differently, and they will be treated differently."

Practice moderation and avoid overtraining. If overuse problems occur, get a professional diagnosis. Cindy Nayer recommends, "Do not wait for persistent pain to set in. Working through pain, however intermittent, is never smart." Allow the body adequate recovery time. If injured, rest the affected area and only begin exercising again after consulting with your exercise leader and/or your doctor. You may need to perform low-impact stretching exercises to help the injury heal.

Cool down properly. Take a minimum of five minutes to gradually decrease your heart rate to near resting level. Utilize general movement patterns similar to the exercises just performed. Include stretching exercises for flexibility enhancement.

Conclusion

Dance exercise injury can be minimized by altering the performance of selected exercises. Learning what puts you at risk is the first step in reducing it. William Vetter and his colleagues report that "provided some restraint is exercised to avoid risky training errors, aerobic dance may well be a safe and enjoyable technique to achieve and maintain aerobic fitness." According to James Garrick, "When viewed from a purely medical perspective, aerobic dance appears to offer well-documented fitness enhancement with a minimum of risk. Perhaps even more important, it has appealed to a large group of women previously uninvolved in any fitness activity. It would be unfortunate if the efforts of the highly vocal detractors serve only to discourage participation by those who are both the most impressionable and most in need of such a program."

GLOSSARY

Achilles tendonitis. Inflammation of the Achilles tendon, which runs from the back of the calf to the heel.

Aerobic exercise. Exercise that works your cardiovascular system, usually consisting of movements that work the large muscle groups (found in the arms or legs) in a repetitive fashion for at least twenty minutes. For optimal gains, you should exercise three to five times a week for twenty to sixty minutes each session.

All-fours. A position in which you support yourself on hands and knees.

Anatomic malalignment. Muscles that are not positioned or bones that don't articulate (fit together) properly. A *functional malalignment* is caused by weak or inflexible muscles, and is treated by muscle strengthening and stretching exercises. A *structural malalignment* (such as bones that don't fit together properly) is treated with orthotics or other aids.

Anterior. Front.

Ballistic exercises. Exercises involving bouncing in a position to stretch the muscles; these should generally be avoided.

Bursa. Liquid-filled pouch that acts as a shock absorber in a joint.

Bursitis. Inflammation of a bursa.

Cartilage. Hard substance that is more flexible than fully developed bone and more rigid than ligament (for example, the end of your nose).

Cool-down. Low-intensity activities, including static stretches, to help the body return to its resting state after a workout. *Compare* Warmup.

Duration. How long you exercise.

Extension. Moving two body segments away from each other. *Compare* Flexion.

Flexion. Moving two body segments toward each other. *Compare* Extension.

Frequency. How often you exercise.

Grand plié. *See plié.*

Hyperextension. Straightening a muscle or joint beyond its normal range, possibly leading to strain or injury. *Compare* Hyperflexion.

Hyperflexion. Bending a muscle or joint beyond normal limits, possibly leading to strain or injury. *Compare* Hyperextension.

Hypervitaminosis. An abnormal state caused by long-term ingestion of excessive vitamins.

Intensity. How hard you exercise.

Isometric exercise. Exercise in which tension is generated in a muscle or group of muscles but no movement occurs (such as when you push against a wall).

Isotonic exercise. Exercise in which the muscle develops tension while moving (such as when you lift weights).

Kyphosis. Rounding (usually of the upper back or shoulders).

Ligament. Connecting tissue that links bone to bone.

Load. Resistance or weight against which a muscle works.

Microtrauma. Small injury to a muscle or connective tissue caused by friction, impact, or overuse.

Myotatic reflex. *See* Stretch reflex.

Orthotic. Insert placed in a shoe to correct an anatomical malalignment or to treat an injury.

Osteoarthritis. Inflammation of bones or joints.

Osteoporosis. Bone loss often associated with calcium deficiencies in older women.

Overload. Subjecting a muscle to greater-than-normal resistance or weight.

Overuse syndrome. The repetitive working of a muscle or muscles without allowing adequate time for recovery, leading to strain or injury. Overuse syndrome can be caused by doing too much too soon, exercising too many days each week, or completing too many repetitions of a movement.

Plantar fasciitis. Inflammation of the plantar fascia, a thick band of tissue running along the base of the foot. The condition is often caused by a collapsed arch, and is the second most common injury in aerobic dance.

Plié. To bend, usually at the knee. In ballet, flexion at the hips, knees, and ankles, usually with the legs turned out, while holding the torso upright. In a *demi-plié*, the heels remain on the floor; while in a *grand plié*, the heels release from the floor, allowing greater flexion at the three joints, resulting in a deeper *plié*.

Posterior. Rear.

Pronation. Rolling in (usually referring to the feet). *See* Supination.

***Pyriformis* syndrome.** Irritation of the *pyriformis* muscle, located deep in the buttocks.

Sciatica. Inflammation along the sciatic nerve. Generally used to describe pain in the buttocks, lower back, hips, or adjacent areas.

Shinsplint. Generic term for pain in the shins or lower legs. This problem is the most common injury in aerobics.

Sportsmedicine. The study of the effects of sports or exercise on your body, and the common injuries that may occur.

Stretch reflex. A muscle that is forcefully stretched elicits a reflex causing it to contract, potentially leading to strain or injury. *Also called* Myotatic reflex.

Subluxation. Partial dislocation of a bone, such as when the upper arm partially pops out of the shoulder joint.

Supination. Rolling out (usually referring to the feet). *See* Pronation.

Tendon. Tissue that connects muscles to bones.

Tendonitis. Inflammation of a tendon.

Torque. Turning or twisting force, or a measurement of the rotational force created by a moving object.

Turnout. Rotation of the leg from the hips. In ballet, a full rotation of the legs resulting in a 90-degree shift of each foot from its normal (full-front) position.

Valsalva maneuver. Any exercise in which you hold your breath while straining.

Vertebrae. The small, ring-shaped bones that make up the spinal column.

Warmup. Pre-exercise workout to loosen up the muscles for activity and increase blood flow and temperature. A typical warmup consists of low-intensity movements (such as walking) and stretches of the same muscles that are to be used in your exercise program. *Compare* Cool-down.

Workload. *See* Load.

RESOURCE LIST

Aerobic & Fitness Association of America (AFAA)
15250 Ventura Blvd., Suite 310
Sherman Oaks, CA 91403
800-446-2322

American Alliance for Health, Physical Education, Recreation and Dance (AAHPERD)
1900 Association Dr.
Reston, VA 22091
703-476-3400

American College of Sports Medicine (ACSM)
401 W. Michigan St.
Indianapolis, IN 46202-3233
317-637-9200

American Council on Exercise (ACE, formerly IDEA)
6190 Conerstone Court East, Suite 202
San Diego, CA 92121-4729
619-535-8227

American Heart Association (AHA)
7320 Greenville Ave.
Dallas, TX 75231
214-373-6300

American Medical Association (AMA)
515 N. State St.
Chicago, IL 60610
312-464-5000

Association for Fitness in Business (AFB)
200 Marott Ctr.
342 Massachusetts Ave.
Indianapolis, IN 46204
317-636-6621

Institute for Aerobics Research
12330 Preston Rd.
Dallas, TX 75230
214-701-8001

International Association for Dance Medicine and Science (IADMS)
4510 West 77th Street, Suite 114
Minneapolis, MN 55435

National Strength and Conditioning Association (NSCA)
300 Old City Hall Landmark
920 O Street
Lincoln, NE 68508
402-472-3000

REFERENCES

ACSM. 1986. *Guidelines for exercise testing and prescription.* 3rd ed. Philadelphia, PA: Lea & Febiger.

———. 1990. The recommended quantity and quality of exercise for developing and maintaining cardiorespiratory and muscular fitness in healthy adults. *Medicine and Science in Sports and Exercise* 22(2): 265-274.

Adrian, M., and J. Cooper. 1989. *The biomechanics of human movement.* Indianapolis, IN: Benchmark Press.

Alan, K. 1987. An injury prevention update. Presentation given at the IDEA Conference, University of Nevada, Reno.

Albohm, M. 1987. Musculoskeletal injuries. In *Aerobic dance-exercise instructor manual,* ed. N. Van Gelder. San Diego, CA: IDEA Foundation.

American Academy of Pediatrics. 1982. Risks in long distance running for children. *The Physician and Sportsmedicine* 10(8): 155–159.

Arnheim, D. 1991. *Dance injuries: Their prevention and care.* 3rd ed. Princeton, NJ: Dance Horizons/Princeton Book Company.

Besson, P. 1987. *Fitness forum.* Newton, MA: Fitness Resource Association.

Brehm, B. 1987. The warm-up: Its physiological contribution to safe and effective exercise. *Fitness Management* 3(6): 19–20.

———. 1988. How to give safe counsel to your pregnant exercisers. *Fitness Management* 4(6): 18–20.

Calhoun, S. 1986. No room for compromising positions. *Dance Exercise Today* 4(1): 26–30.

Casten, C., and P. Jordan. 1990. *Aerobics today.* St. Paul, MN: West Publishing.

Clippinger-Robertson, K. 1987. Components of an aerobic dance-exercise class. In *Aerobic dance-exercise instructor manual,* ed. N. Van Gelder. San Diego, CA.: IDEA Foundation.

———. 1988. Understanding contraindicated exercises. *Dance Exercise Today* 6(1): 57-60.

Corbin, C., and R. Lindsey. 1988. *Concepts of physical fitness with laboratories.* 6th ed. Dubuque, IA: Wm. C. Brown.

Ellison, D. 1987. Exercise technique: Correct hip exercises. *Dance Exercise Today* 5(2): 22-23.

Eoff, N. L., and D. Q. Thomas. 1987. Exercise videos: A critical analysis. *Fitness in Business* 1(5): 179-183.

Francis, P., and L. Francis. 1986. Injury prevention: The hip and lower back. *Dance Exercise Today* 4(2): 27.

———. 1986. Injury prevention: Defining contraindicated exercises. *Dance Exercise Today* 3(4): 22.

Francis, L., P. Francis, and K. Welshons-Smith. 1985. Aerobic dance injuries: A survey of instructors. *The Physician and Sportsmedicine* 13(2): 105-111.

Garrick, J. 1987. Aerobic dance injuries and their prevention. In *Dance medicine: A comprehensive guide,* ed. A. Ryan and R. Stephens. Chicago, IL and Minneapolis, MN: Pluribus Press and *The Physician and Sportsmedicine.*

———. 1989. Anterior knee pain (chondromalacia patellae). *The Physician and Sportsmedicine* 17(1): 75-83.

Gettman, L. 1988. Fitness testing. In *Resource manual for guidelines for exercise testing and prescription.* Philadelphia, PA: Lea & Febiger.

Goodman, C. 1987. Case reports: Low back pain in the cosmetic athlete. *The Physician and Sportsmedicine* 15(8): 97-102.

Kannel, W. B., D. McGee, and T. Gordon. 1976. A general cardiovascular risk profile: The Framingham study. *American Journal of Cardiology* 38: 46-51.

Kelly, E. 1987. The dancer's back. *JOPERD* 58(5): 41-44.

Kravitz, L., and S. Kutner. 1988. Exercise technique: Training the abdominals. *Dance Exercise Today* 6(8): 25-26.

Kravitz, S. 1987. Basic concepts of biomechanics: Relating the foot and ankle to overuse injuries. *JOPERD* 58(5): 31-33.

Kreighbaum, E. 1987. Anatomy and kinesiology. In *Aerobic dance-exercise instructors manual,* ed. N. Van Gelder. San Diego, CA: IDEA Foundation.

Lehman, B. 1989. Unfit for exercise. *The Boston Globe* (Oct. 23): 25-26.

Lindsey, R., and C. Corbin. 1989. Questionable exercises—some safer alternatives. *JOPERD* 60(8): 26-32.

Lubell, A. 1989. Potentially dangerous exercises: Are they harmful to all? *The Physician and Sportsmedicine* 17(1): 187-192.

Memory jogger: Exercises to prevent and treat low back pain. *The Physician and Sportsmedicine* 15(1): 116.

Micheli, L. (1988). Overuse injuries: Etiology and assessment. Paper presented at the New England Chapter of the American College of Sportsmedicine Convention, Worcester, MA.

National Strength and Conditioning Association. 1985. Position paper on prepubescent strength training. *National Strength and Conditioning Association Journal* 7(4): 27-31.

Nayer, C. 1987. Injury prevention: Prevent overtraining. *Dance Exercise Today* 5(3): 44.

Norris, R. 1987. Dance doctor. *Dance Umbrella Newsletter* 2(3): 3.

———. 1987. Dance doctor. *Dance Umbrella Newsletter* 2(4): 3.

O'Brien, S., and P. Vertinsky. 1991. Unfit survivors: Exercise as a resource for aging women. *Gerontologist* 31(3): 347-357.

Ocker, G. 1987. See which shoes stand up to our expert's scrutiny. *Shape* (Sept.): 113-114.

Pangrazi, R., and V. Dauer. 1992. *Dynamic physical education for elementary school children*. 10th ed. NY: Macmillan.

Richie, D., S. Kelso, and P. Bellucci. 1985. Aerobic dance injuries: A retrospective study of instructors and participants. *The Physician and Sportsmedicine* 13(2): 130-140.

Rikli, R. and D. Edwards. 1991. Effects of a three-year exercise program on motor function and cognitive processing speed in older women. *Research Quarterly for Exercise and Sport* 62(1): 61-67.

Ryan, N. 1989. Preventing participant dropout: Guidelines for dance exercise instructors, program directors, and club owners. *In Critical issues in HPER: A global analysis*. Frostburg, MD.: Proceedings from the 32nd Anniversary World Congress, International Council for Health, Physical Education, Recreation, and Dance.

Smith, K. 1988. Train don't strain: A guide to safe and effective exercise. *Journal of the Maryland AHPERD* (Winter): 24-26.

———. 1987. Effective exercise. *Journal of the Maryland AHPERD* (Spring): 2-3.

———. 1987. Getting started with exercise. *Go Magazine* (Spring): 2-3.

Smith, L. 1988. Health appraisal. In *Resource manual for guidelines for exercise testing and prescription*. Philadelphia, PA: Lea & Febiger.

Solomon, R., and L. Micheli. 1986. Technique as a consideration in modern dance injuries. *The Physician and Sportsmedicine* 14(8): 83-89.

Stone, W. 1987. *Adult fitness programs.* Glenview, IL: Scott, Foresman.

Teitz, C. 1987. Patellofemoral pain in dancers. *JOPERD* 58(5): 34-36.

Thomas, D. Q., and N. Rippee. 1988. Selecting an exercise video. *Fitness in Business* (August): 12-15.

Timmermans, H., and M. Martin. 1987. Top ten potentially dangerous exercises. *JOPERD* 58(6): 29-32.

Vetter, W., D. Helfet, K. Spear, and L. Matthews. 1985. Aerobic dance injuries. *The Physician and Sportsmedicine* 13(2): 114-120.

Wallace, J. 1987. Exercise and pregnancy: Physiological considerations. In *Aerobic dance-exercise instructors manual,* ed. N. Van Gelder. San Diego, CA: IDEA Foundation.

Wells, C. 1991. *Women, sport, and performance.* 2nd ed. Champaign, IL: Human Kinetics.

Winden, K. 1990. Exercise guidelines for pregnancy. Paper presented at the meeting of the Southwest District Association for Health, Physical Education, Recreation, and Dance, Albuquerque, NM.

Work, J. 1989. Strength training: A bridge to independence. *The Physician and Sportsmedicine* 17(11): 134-140.

Zebas, C. 1987. Exercise safety for abdominal strengthening. *Certified* 2(1): 18-19.

ADDITIONAL REFERENCES

Aerobics and Fitness Association of America. 1985. *Aerobics: Theory and Practice.* Sherman Oaks: AFAA.

Alter, Judy. 1983. *Surviving exercise.* Boston: Houghton Mifflin.

———. 1986. *Stretch and strengthen.* Boston: Houghton Mifflin.

Berardi, Gigi. 1991. *Finding balance: Fitness and training for a lifetime in dance.* Princeton, NJ: Dance Horizons/Princeton Book Company.

Caillet, René. 1984. *Understand your backache: A guide to prevention, treatment, and relief.* Philadelphia, PA: F.A. Davis.

Chmelar, Robin D., and Sally S. Fitt. 1990. *Dancing at your peak: Diet, A complete guide to nutrition and weight control.* Princeton, NJ: Dance Horizons/Princeton Book Company.

Clarkson, Priscilla M., and Margaret Skrinar, eds. 1988. *Science of dance training.* Champaign, IL: Human Kinetics.

Featherstone, D. F. 1970. *Dancing without danger: A guide to the prevention of injury for the amateur and professional dancer.* NY: A. S. Barnes.

Franks, B. Don, and Edward T. Howley. 1989. *Fitness Leader's Handbook.* Champaign, IL: Human Kinetics.

Horosko, Marian, and J. R. F. Kupersmith. 1987. *The dancer's survival manual.* NY: Harper & Row.

Howse, A. J. G., and S. Hancock. 1988. *Dance technique and injury prevention.* NY: Theatre Arts Books.

Kenney, W. Larry, ed. 1992. *American College of Sports Medicine Fitness Book.* Champaign, IL: Leisure Press.

Kent, Allegra, with James and Constance Camner. 1984. *The dancer's body book.* NY: William Morrow.

Mazzeo, Karen S. 1992. *Aerobic Dance—A Way to Fitness.* 3rd ed. Englewood, CO: Morton Publishing Co.

Nagrin, Daniel. 1988. *How to dance forever: Surviving against the odds.* NY: William Morrow.

Paskevska, Anna. 1992. *Both sides of the mirror: The science and art of ballet.* 2nd ed. Princeton, NJ: Dance Horizons/Princeton Book Company.

Ryan, Allan J., and Robert E. Stephens, eds. 1987. *Dance medicine: A comprehensive guide.* Chicago, IL: Pluribus Press.

———. 1988. *The dancer's complete guide to healthcare and a long career.* Chicago, IL: Bonus Books.

Shell, Caroline G., ed. 1986. *The dancer as athlete.* Champaign, IL: Human Kinetics.

Spilken, Terry L. 1990. *The dancer's foot book: A complete guide to foot care.* Princeton, NJ: Dance Horizons/Princeton Book Company.

Vincent, L. M. 1978. *The dancer's book of health.* Princeton, NJ: Dance Horizons/Princeton Book Company.

———. 1989. *Competing with the sylph.* 2nd ed. Princeton, NJ: Dance Horizons/Princeton Book Company.

Watkins, Andrea, and Priscilla M. Clarkson. 1990. *Dancing longer, dancing stronger: A dancer's guide to improving technique and preventing injury.* Princeton, NJ: Dance Horizons/Princeton Book Company.

Wilmoth, Susan K. 1986. *Leading Aerobic Dance-Exercise.* Champaign, IL: Human Kinetics.

Wright, Stuart. 1985. *Dancer's guide to injuries of the lower extremities.* Cranbury, NJ: Cornwall Books.

Index

C

D-E

F-G

H-I